"BASED ON THE THEORY THAT YOUR MEMORY CAN BE EXERCISED LIKE ANY OTHER PART OF A TIME-AFFECTED BODY, THIS BOOK OFFERS SIMPLE WAYS TO INCREASE YOUR LONG-TERM AND SHORT-TERM MEMORY."—*American Way*

## WHIP YOUR MEMORY INTO SHAPE TODAY!

In this remarkable book, Dr. Cynthia Green outlines her simple and effective program to achieve maximum memory fitness in just eight easy lessons. Each lesson focuses on one aspect of memory followed by a series of specific "memorcises" designed to build memory muscle.

### Inside you'll find fun and effective ways to:
- Remember names and faces
- Recall important information at work
- Improve your retention of facts in books and technical data
- Keep track of appointments and dates
- Remember where you put your keys, left your glasses, parked your car

### You'll also learn:
- The ten lifestyle factors most likely to lower your memory—and how to change them
- The best diet to boost your brain power
- The truth about "memory enhancing" supplements such as gi
- How certain medic affect memory perfo
- When memory lapses are they may indicate an underlying disease
- And much more!

# TOTAL MEMORY WORKOUT

## 8 Easy Steps to Maximum Memory Fitness

## Cynthia R. Green, Ph.D.

*Director of The Memory Enhancement Program
at Mount Sinai School of Medicine*

Bantam Books
New York   Toronto   London
Sydney   Auckland

TOTAL MEMORY WORKOUT

PUBLISHING HISTORY
Bantam hardcover / September 1999
Bantam trade paperback / February 2001

Grateful acknowledgment for reprinting the following excerpts:
On pages 69–70 from *Little House in the Big Woods* by Laura Ingalls Wilder. Text copyright © 1932 by Laura Ingalls Wilder; copyright renewed © 1959 by Roger Lea MacBride. Used by permission of HarperCollins Publishers, Inc. "Little House"® is a registered trademark of HarperCollins Publishers, Inc. On page 172 from article "Singapore Limits Its Vehicle Population," from the July 1997 issue of *Automotive Engineering*. Reprinted with permission SAE Automotive Engineering. Copyright © 1997 by Society of Automotive Engineers, Inc. All rights reserved.

*Book design by Jennifer Ann Daddio.*

Library of Congress Catalog Card Number: 99-30960

ISBN 0-553-38026-5

*Published simultaneously in the United States and Canada*

Bantam Books are published by Bantam Books, a division of Random House, Inc. Its trademark, consisting of the words "Bantam Books" and the portrayal of a rooster, is Registered in U.S. Patent and Trademark Office and in other countries. Marca Registrada. Bantam Books, 1540 Broadway, New York, New York 10036.

PRINTED IN THE UNITED STATES OF AMERICA

(BVG)   10

*To Joshua, Zachary, and Jonah*
*with whom I share my most special memories*

# Contents

# Acknowledgments

There are many people I wish to acknowledge for their support during this project. I would like to thank my mentor and colleague, Dr. Richard Mohs, for the opportunity to continue his initial explorations into memory improvement as well as for the confidence and support he has given me throughout my career. I am grateful as well to my department chairman, Dr. Kenneth Davis, who allowed me the freedom to explore and develop an area of work not typically within the activities of our department; and to Dr. Deborah Marin, for her professional and personal support as well as her friendship.

The program presented here is based not only on my experiences in teaching memory effectiveness but also on the observations of my students. I am grateful to all my "alumni" who have helped me fine-tune my professional knowledge about memory improvement into information that real people can use. Thank you as well to my colleagues Anne Peterson and Tracy Lippes, who in learning how to teach with me were able to collaborate on making the program better. I am grateful for the help provided by Dr. Rosemarie Bria, particularly in Step 3. I also would like to acknowledge Jill Smith for her able assistance.

Thank you to my agent, Pam Bernstein, for helping me

recognize the potential for this book and for her invaluable guidance every step along the way; and to Donna Downing, who always seems to know the answer whenever a question arises. I am grateful to the staff of Bantam Books who have been so dedicated to making this book come to life. Robin Michaelson proved to be not only a goddess of the written word but also a true collaborator. Thank you, Robin, for making this such a wonderful experience. Special thanks as well to Toni Burbank for shepherding the project through so smoothly, to Jean Lynch for her keen copyediting eye, and to Betsy Hulsebosch and Barb Burg for their help.

The support of my family and friends was invaluable in making this book a reality. I am especially grateful to my parents, Susan and Ronald Green, for teaching me that I could do anything I wanted to do if I only tried; and to my grandmothers, Florence Green and Charlotte Falk, for setting such wonderful examples. Thank you as well to Judy and Stephen Peck for their support; to Beverly Jablons for extending to me the same unequivocable backing she gives Josh; and to all my siblings, by blood and marriage, for their encouragement. A special thank you to Elsie Macedonio for loving my boys so much. I am thankful as well for the unending generosity of my friends, who have tolerated me with such good humor during this process. Thank you in particular to Adine Duron and Durston Saylor.

I have the good fortune of being married to my best friend. This book is in no small part the result of Josh's belief in what I could do and his prodding me to do it. Thank you, best buddy, for encouraging me to pursue my dreams, for your support even when it wasn't easy, and for the time you gave me to write. Finally, a big thank you to Zach and Jonah for being the two most wonderful boys in the whole world. You always help Mommy remember what's really important.

# TOTAL MEMORY WORKOUT

# Introduction

*"It is not enough to have a good mind.*
*The main thing is to use it well."*
— RENÉ DESCARTES

What did you forget today? Perhaps it was your keys as you were
walking out the door. Maybe it was an important conference call,
a permission slip for your child's field trip next week, or a stop at
the dry cleaners. Chances are, whoever you are, you forgot something you wish you'd remembered.

Forgetting is part of being human. All of us forget, no matter
how young we are, no matter how many balls we juggle. Perhaps
you have noticed changes in your memory as you've grown older
and are feeling a bit anxious about them. Maybe you have more
responsibilities at work, young children at home, and are finding it
hard to keep track of everything you have to do. Concern about
how well we remember knows no age limit. Memory fitness is a
hot topic for everyone, from professionals in their twenties deter-
mined to get ahead at work and working parents with young children who fear that the kids are eating their brain cells, to baby
boomers who are worried about keeping up and recent retirees who
want to enjoy their new pursuits to the fullest.

Even though it may be normal to forget from time to time, it's still frustrating when we can't remember when we really *need* to. Can we remember better? Absolutely. For the past several years, I have been teaching people how to achieve maximum memory fitness. I am a clinical psychologist who has specialized in memory function and memory disorders for many years. Over time, my colleagues and I found that we were seeing a larger number of people who were perfectly healthy yet worried about their memory. While we could reassure them that nothing was seriously wrong with their ability to remember, we found that there was little practical information available to help people understand and improve their memory health and wellness. The Memory Enhancement Program at Mount Sinai School of Medicine in New York City was established in response to this growing need.

As founder and director of this program, I have had the opportunity to develop a unique memory wellness series designed specifically for healthy individuals interested in improving their memory. This course has already helped hundreds of healthy adults of all ages learn simple but powerful ways to boost their brainpower. My clients come from all walks of life—they are busy professionals, real estate agents, firefighters, soccer moms, artists, lawyers, musicians, retirees. A thirty-three-year-old film producer comes to improve his memory skills so he can be more effective at work. A ninety-one-year-old grandmother attends because she is anxious to be better at remembering lines for her acting class. What all my clients have in common is that they are all active, involved individuals who want to make the most of their memory. In other words, they are just like you.

*Total Memory Workout* allows you to benefit from this unique training just as if you were working with me personally or attending one of my seminars. Drawing on my expertise as a memory specialist, I will teach you:

- How memory works—and how it doesn't.
- How factors in your daily lifestyle, such as fatigue, medications, and stress, can lower your memory potential, along with advice on how to minimize their impact.
- The pros and cons of current medical interventions for memory improvement, including hormone replacement therapy, vitamin supplementation, and herbal remedies.
- The best way to use memory tools, such as appointment books, calendars, and checklists, so they *really* work for you.
- Practical techniques for remembering information that you read in books or newspapers, or see in shows or movies.
- Simple steps you can take to boost your brainpower in remembering names.

You will find that *Total Memory Workout* is very different from other books on memory. What makes this book unique? After all, memory improvement programs have been around for many years. Other memory experts teach difficult, cumbersome techniques for people who want "super" memories. Such complex memory systems can be effective, but they require too much time to master and use to be of interest to the average person. To tell you the truth, I rarely meet people who want to remember the names of everyone in a crowd of two hundred people. In other words, such methods can work, but can they really work for *you*?

*Total Memory Workout* uses a memory wellness approach. You will learn that memory is not merely an intellectual skill to be manipulated, but rather an integral part of ourselves, affected by many aspects of our daily lives. This book will teach you *all* about memory, from the basics of how we acquire and remember information to what elements in our lifestyles can lower memory potential. You will be trained in memory techniques that are easy to learn and that you can really use. I will teach you simple methods that you can instantly fit into your lifestyle and adopt as good memory habits to enhance your memory effectiveness. Several alternative techniques will be offered in the program's steps, so that you can find the ones that work best for you. There is no single right way or best way to improve your memory. We all need to find out what works for us and—most importantly—use it.

## The Best Way to Use This Book

Years of teaching folks how to remember better has given me some experience in the best way to approach memory improvement. Here's some advice for getting the most out of this program:

• **Read each step.** *Total Memory Workout* is divided into eight steps, or lessons. Read one step at a time. While I recommend going through them in order, it is possible to skip around to particular topics of interest. These steps build on each other, but they are also self-contained. So, if you have a dinner party next week and want to rev up your recall for names, go right ahead to Step 7, "Remember the People You Meet."

• **Focus on one step per week.** You will get the most out of this book by doing one step per week. This will give you time to master and practice your new memory habits. Also, pacing yourself in learning information gives your brain time to consolidate it. Like a good exercise regimen or a good diet, this program works best when you incorporate these techniques into your daily routine and really use them.

• **Take the quizzes.** At the end of each step is a short quiz. Make sure you do the quizzes so you can see how much you remember!

• **Do the Memorcises.** Each lesson is followed by exercises, or what I call "Memorcises." The Memorcises give you a chance to practice what you have been taught. *It is very important that you do the Memorcises.* You cannot fully benefit from this program if you do not use the methods taught here. Making the work personal is especially important, since my approach gives you many ways to improve your memory fitness, and with that freedom comes the responsibility of determining your own private memory prescription. The Memorcises allow you to "test-drive" the techniques and figure out how to make this program work for you.

• **Relax and enjoy it.** This is the most important thing you can do to benefit from this unique training program. Having fun while you train your brain will make it easier to achieve maximum memory fitness.

# STEP
## 1

# Meet Your Memory

■ IN THIS STEP YOU WILL LEARN: ■

*Favorite Fallacies About Memory*
*How Memory Works*
*How Memory Can Change as We Age*
*What Doesn't Change*
*Wake Up Your Memory with the A.M. Principle*

## Favorite Fallacies About Memory

How do you think memory works? While most of us have some idea about how we learn and remember information, there are some things we may believe that simply are not true. In teaching memory improvement over the years, I have frequently been asked questions that show me that people have been misled about their memory, often in ways that cause them unnecessary worry. Let's go over some of my favorite fallacies about memory.

### THE "SECRET HANDSHAKE" FALLACY
Do you believe that there are people who have a great memory because they have access to some secret that allows them to

remember everything and forget nothing? If only you too could learn that secret handshake! The truth is, *there is no secret to having a good memory.* A good memory is the result of good habits and practice, practice, practice. Better memory fitness is something that *anyone* can have.

## THE "EASY STREET" FALLACY

Some of the same people who believe that there's a secret to having a good memory also feel that once you know this magic formula, it's easy to remember. Would you be surprised to learn that life on memory lane is no easy street? There's no quick and simple trick for improving your memory. If you want a healthier memory, you must better your overall memory fitness. And like anything else in life that's worth having, a good memory is the result of work. Even people who seem to have super memory powers must work at remembering. Of course, better memory habits become easier to keep as you incorporate them into your daily routine. Think about this: Do you brush your teeth? Yes. Were you born knowing how to brush your teeth? Of course not. You learned this healthy habit and now don't even think twice about it. You can learn better memory habits and make them as much a part of your life as brushing your teeth.

## THE "MEMORY CURE" FALLACY

Some people feel that they don't really need to work on improving their memory, since someone will soon come up with a magic pill they can take that will "fix" their memory for them. Given the hype about so many of these so-called memory cures, it's hard to blame them for feeling this way. In fact, the memory remedy field has become quite a big business. It is estimated that in 1997 Americans spent $90.2 million on ginkgo biloba, an herbal supplement reputed to boost memory. The claims made by many of the manufacturers of these supplements are, well, unbelievable. My favorite is a flyer I received in the mail touting the incredible feats of a special tonic, which stated in large bold letters that "scientists discover that age spots signal the start of senility, but there's a way to deter them, and dramatically improve your health at the same time." How can you keep yourself from "going senile"? By using— what else?—this special tonic.

*There is no such thing as a "memory cure" for your memory.* For most of us, our memory isn't sick or broken. It doesn't need to be cured—we just need to get it into shape. Also, while some of these supplements may be beneficial, many of the claims made on their behalf are not supported by scientific evidence. In Step 3 I'll discuss which supplements you may want to consider taking, as well as those which may be a waste of your money. But you will never achieve maximum memory fitness by taking a pill. Even if you find a supplement helpful, your memory will not improve significantly unless you also make better memory habits part of your lifestyle.

## THE "MEMORY SUPERHERO" FALLACY

Meet our memory superhero. With his well developed memory muscles and superior strength, he remembers everything, including where he has left his keys at all times, every errand his wife has asked him to run, *and* all birthdays and anniversaries. Hopefully, you are old enough now to realize that superheroes don't exist. Memory lapses are part of the normal human experience. Even memory improvement experts forget from time to time. The goal of improving your memory shouldn't be to have perfect recall—that just isn't realistic. Wanting to remember better, though, is a reasonable expectation we can have of ourselves. People who remember better practice good memory habits, habits that you too can learn.

There are, of course, those rare individuals who do have superior memories. It is estimated that about one in a million adults has eidetic or photographic memory ability. This doesn't mean that these people remember absolutely everything. Instead, they have incredible power to recall visually mediated information. A "perfect" memory is even rarer. One such case was S., a mnemonist, or memory performer, who was carefully studied over many years by the famous neurologist A. R. Luria. In his fascinating book *The Mind of a Mnemonist: A Little Book About a Vast Memory*, Luria reported in detail on the nature of S.'s memory. S. not only had the uncanny ability to recollect perfectly everything that had been said to him recently, but he could also remember in detail conversations held several years earlier. S. had what is known as *synesthesia*—he not only heard something, but also saw it and tasted it. Thus, his memories were associated with colors, shapes, sounds, and tastes. However, this perfect memory did not make for a happy life. S. had, as Luria describes, great difficulty pursuing a "normal" existence:

> An individual whose conscious awareness is such that a sound becomes fused with a sense of color and taste; for whom each fleeting impression engenders a vivid, inextinguishable image; for whom words have quite different meanings than they do for us—such a person cannot mature in the same way others do, nor will his inner world, his life history, tend to be like others'. A person who has "seen" and experienced life synesthetically cannot have the same grasp of things the rest of us have, nor is he likely to experience himself or other people as we might.[1]

[1] A. R. Luria, *The Mind of a Mnemonist: A Little Book About a Vast Memory* (Cambridge: Harvard University Press, 1968), p. 151.

Reading about S. always reminds me of the saying "Be careful what you wish for, you may get it." We don't need to be memory superheroes to have memories that work well for us.

## THE "IF IT'S BROKE, YOU CAN'T FIX IT" FALLACY

How often have you heard someone complain that they have never had a good memory? I hear this all the time. Some people feel that they have always had a hard time remembering names, lists, or anything at all. Perhaps you feel this way yourself.

The truth is, there is no such thing as a "bad" memory. Memory is not a one-dimensional process. Rather, it is a complex, multidimensional function with many facets, including odors, sounds, tastes, sight, and language. Just as we have strengths and weaknesses in physical ability, we have strengths and weaknesses in different areas of memory. For example, maybe you have a great visual memory and tend to remember things very well if you've seen them or if you can picture them. But the person next to you on the bus may have a very good aural memory, remembering things that they hear. An example is my client, Carol T.*:

*A successful composer and performer in her fifties, Carol T. came to my memory enhancement class when she began to forget more often where she'd put things or errands she had to run. The changes were really just irritating to her, but she became especially frustrated when she started to forget lyrics she had thought of and planned to write down later. In the first class, as we discussed individual strengths and weaknesses in memory functioning, Carol realized that because of her strong memory for sound, she never had the same difficulty recalling music she had composed in her head as she did recalling lyrics.*

* Names of the case study subjects mentioned in this book have been changed to protect their privacy.

Just because you have strengths in an area of memory doesn't mean that the rest of your memory is "bad." Most healthy people who complain about having a poor memory simply have never been taught the skills necessary for good memory fitness. Unfortunately, this is not true for people who suffer from an underlying disease that causes changes in memory, or who have experienced an injury that has made it more difficult for them to remember. However, even these individuals can be helped by taking some simple steps to make the most of their remaining memory power.

## THE "OLD GEEZER" FALLACY

Many people believe that losing your memory is just another part of growing older. Today we know that *serious memory loss is not an inevitable consequence of aging,* but the result of disease. While it is true that you are at increased risk for a dementia, such as Alzheimer's disease, as you grow older, the risk is lower than many people believe. While we can experience mild changes in memory as we age, these changes do not necessarily mean we are suffering from a disease that will progressively worsen. As Drs. John Rowe and Robert Kahn note in their seminal book *Successful Aging,* "The view that old age is inevitably accompanied by substantial reductions in mental function is clearly wrong. . . . Growing old, for most people, means maintaining full mental functions."[2]

Even if you experience some mild changes in your memory as you grow older, it is possible that you won't be troubled by them. What bothers us most, after all, depends on what we value about ourselves. Some of us may be more upset by the gray hair and wrinkles that come along with aging than we are by changes in memory. A professional athlete may be more distressed by physical changes that happen as she ages, and may care less about not being able to remember words as well. A writer or lawyer, on the other

[2] J. W. Rowe and R. L. Kahn, *Successful Aging* (New York: Pantheon Books, 1998), p. 91.

> *"There is a wicked inclination in most people to suppose an old man decayed in his intellects. If a young or middle-aged man, when leaving company, does not recollect where he laid his hat, it is nothing; but if the same inattention is discovered in an old man, people will shrug up their shoulders and say, 'His memory is going.'"*
> —SAMUEL JOHNSON

hand, may be very frustrated by difficulty finding words, but not at all concerned that he can't run as quickly as when he was younger. The good news for those of us who *are* bothered by changes in our memory is that although they are annoying, these changes do not deter people from leading active, productive lives. Research has shown that you can maximize your memory potential no matter what your age by learning to cope effectively with the changes you may experience. You are never too old—or too young—to learn how to rev up your recall.

## How Memory Works

Now that we have dispelled some popular fallacies about memory, how does memory really work? As you might imagine, memory function is rather complex and the object of much research. Luckily, you need to know only the basics of how memory operates to help you move forward in making yours more fit. So let's go ahead and meet your memory.

### THE THREE STEPS OF MEMORY

How we learn and remember is a subject that has always greatly intrigued scientists. Current memory theorists generally consider memory as requiring three steps: acquisition, storage, and retrieval.

### Acquisition

The first step of memory involves learning the material to be remembered. If information is not acquired, it cannot be stored and recalled at a later time. Acquisition requires attention and focus. As a result, it is *very* sensitive to interference. As we shall see later, most of us have difficulty at this step. Often what we think we forgot, we really didn't "get" in the beginning.

### Storage

After you learn something, it must be stored so that you can remember it later when you need it. An intricate part of the memory process, storage involves "placing" information in the right "location." However, we can determine how we store information so that we'll be more likely to find it and recall it.

### Retrieval

Retrieval is the step of memory that truly involves remembering. Here, we recall information that we previously acquired and stored.

If you think of your memory as a library, you'll see how these steps of memory work. A well run library must *acquire* books or other materials. The librarian then must *store* the materials in a meaningful way so they can easily be located and *retrieved* when they are needed. Like a library, your memory must acquire information for future use, sort and organize that information into appropriate storage "locations" so it can be easily found, and retrieve the desired information later when needed.

## THE TWO PROCESSES OF MEMORY

In addition to the steps we use to remember information, we rely on two mechanisms for processing information we need to recall: working memory and long-term memory.

### The Smell of Her Perfume . . .

Why are certain memories crystal clear for us, while other events never even register? The smell of a lover's perfume, the look on a child's face when she takes her first step, the sound of a parent's voice—all are examples of things we may remember as if they happened yesterday. Chances are we really "got" these memories because they happened at a time when our attention was completely engaged, allowing us to capture them quite well. You can help yourself hold on to important moments by consciously focusing your attention when they are happening. Somehow this is still more pleasurable than having them on videotape.

### *Working Memory: The Brain's Scratch Pad*

Working memory, or short-term memory, is generally thought of as the number of information items that can be held in memory for a brief period of time. I often tell people to think of their working memory as a scratch pad for their brain. Working memory is where we "note" information from the world around us. Some of that information we may save, while some of it we will discard.

Working memory is an essential part of our overall memory function. It is the process we use to acquire information we wish to recall. It also allows us to maintain our current picture of the world around us and to keep track of goals or plans we are following at the moment, such as our place in a conversation. However, working memory does have its soft spots. First, there's a limit to how much information we can hold in working memory at any given time. Research has demonstrated our working memory capacity to be five to nine pieces of information. For example, think of a phone number:

## 261-4029

A phone number is seven digits, the average amount of information you can hold in your working memory. But aren't we all able to handle more than that? After all, you may be thinking that you can remember a phone number with its area code using working memory. How does this happen? Well, we naturally tend to take full advantage of our working memory by "chunking," or grouping, information so that we can take it all in. Let's say we need to remember the following address:

**Mr. U. R. Marvelous**
**777 Memory Lane**
**Apt. 222**
**Candotown, MI 25252**

This address contains forty-eight numbers and letters and eleven words or number groups. Either way, it looks theoretically like too much for the typical working memory to retain. Yet we know that we can learn it. How? Our working memory chunks the information together so that it falls at or under the magical number of seven, as follows:

**Chunk 1: name (Mr. U. R. Marvelous)**
**Chunk 2: street address (777 Memory Lane)**
**Chunk 3: apartment (Apt. 222)**
**Chunk 4: town (Candotown)**
**Chunk 5: state (MI)**
**Chunk 6: zip code (25252)**

Working memory capacity varies slightly from person to person. We also know that it can be expanded through attention-building

### *How Strong Are Your Working Memory Muscles?*

How much information can you hold in your working memory? While our memory isn't made of muscle, we know that we can strengthen our working memory by repeated practice, just as an athlete might build muscle strength. Here's a quick way to measure what your working memory can hold.

Below are several strings of numbers. Read the first string of numbers to yourself, then look away and see if you can repeat them in order. Then move on to the next string of numbers. See how many numbers you can remember this way without making a mistake. Remember, the average person can hold from five to nine "chunks" of information in working memory at any given time.

8293

27136

739285

1673820

90461257

528617403

3209861547

05812459306

382749562860

How well did you do?

exercises. As we shall see later, strengthening our working memory muscles by increasing our attention ability is a very important way in which we can boost our brainpower.

Another weakness of working memory is its short-term nature: We don't hold on to information in working memory for very long. Finally, working memory is quite vulnerable to disruption. Chances are you've experienced this when you've lost your train of thought during conversation, or gone into a room to get something and then forgotten what you were looking for. Usually this happens because you were distracted and "lost" that thought or plan from your working memory scratch pad.

Are the limitations of working memory a problem? Of course not. Actually, our working memory is a wonderful intellectual tool that allows us to be flexible and current in our thinking. Just imagine if working memory held on to all the information you got: The world around you would be a jumble. However, we can boost our brainpower by making our working memory more effective so we absorb information better.

### Long-Term Memory

The second process of memory is long-term memory. Long-term memory acts as storage for information we must retain over a greater period of time. This is where we "keep" episodic information, such as what we ate for dinner last night, or what we wore yesterday, so that we don't wear it again today. We also maintain encyclopedic information in long-term memory. Encyclopedic information is material that has been learned very well and stored, such as information learned in school. Long-term memory has a virtually unlimited capacity and is not as easily disrupted as working memory. While certain aspects of daily life can interfere with how well our long-term memory works, in general long-term memory function is relatively insensitive to disruption from the comings and goings of our days.

Many people ask me why they can recall the name of their sixth-grade teacher (are you thinking of that right now?) but not a doc-

*How Long Is Your Long-Term Memory?*

Just how powerful is your long-term memory? Try this simple test: Write down from memory the names of the fifty U.S. states. It doesn't matter how you think of them: alphabetically, geographically, by area code. Just write down as many as you can recall.

Done? How did you do? Chances are you did pretty well, especially if you were born and educated in this country. And when was the last time you wrote down the names of the fifty states? For most of us, it was in grade school. This exercise is a great way to show yourself just how powerful your long-term memory really is.

tor's appointment they made last week. Most likely, the name of your sixth-grade teacher is in your long-term memory, and therefore is easier to recall than an appointment you recently made and to which you may not have paid much attention. You may often surprise yourself with the information you can recall from long-term memory.

So there you have it—all you need to know about how your memory works so you can begin to improve yours. Before we go on, however, let's review what changes in memory we may experience as part of the aging process.

## How Memory Can Change as We Age

How can our memory change as we age? Researchers have documented declines in memory and other intellectual abilities in studies conducted both across different age groups and in individuals followed over time. Many of us begin to experience some changes in memory function around age fifty. What happens?

• **It's harder to learn new things.** As we age, it becomes more difficult for us to learn new information. Does this mean that we *can't* learn anything new? Of course not. For example, my eighty-five-year-old grandmother recently mastered the computer. She now routinely communicates with her nine grandchildren by e-mail, and she also makes on-line purchases. She's typical of older Americans today, many of whom are enthusiastically pursuing brain-building activities, such as taking college classes or traveling. Think how much *you* are able to learn every day. What this does mean, however, is that it may take you additional practice to retain information effectively as you grow older. How can you do that? Simply by developing the better memory habits you will learn in this book.

• **It's harder to focus attention on what's important to remember.** As we grow older, we may have more difficulty directing our attention to information that we want to remember. Researchers have found that our ability to focus and sustain attention decreases with age. It remains unclear why this is the case. The change may be due in part to physiological changes in vision and hearing. Also, older folks tend to use more medications, some of which may have the unintended side effect of interfering with attention. We will discuss lifestyle factors that may decrease attention and lower memory performance in Step 2. However, it just may be that decreased attention is part of growing older. In fact, many researchers have suggested that the memory changes seen in aging are more likely due to these attentional shifts than to any true change in the ability to learn or retrieve information.

Aging may also cause us to have more difficulty multitasking,

### *"When Should I Worry?"*

Only about 15 percent of adults age sixty-five and over develop a degenerative memory disorder such as Alzheimer's disease. However, many people, especially as they age, become concerned that their memory lapses are a sign that they are developing a serious memory problem. As an expert in memory, I am often asked how one can determine whether memory changes are just part of growing older or a sign that something more is happening. I usually offer the following guidelines to help someone decide how serious a problem they are having:

- *Has your memory gotten progressively worse over a period of time, such as six months?*

- *Does your forgetfulness get in the way of your performance at work or make it difficult for you to manage at home with your finances, hobbies, or other activities?*

- *Are your family and friends also worried about what these memory changes mean?*

If you answer yes to these questions, you should consider seeing a health care professional with expertise in memory functioning, such as a geriatrician, neurologist, psychiatrist, or psychologist. Appropriate evaluation of any significant change in memory functioning is always important. Keep in mind that increased forgetfulness is only a symptom. Numerous conditions can cause memory changes, and many of them are treatable.

or dividing our attention among a number of tasks. Dr. Robin West and her colleagues demonstrated this in an experiment in which younger and older adults were given telephone numbers to remember and then were interrupted. They found that the older subjects were much more sensitive to the interference and were more likely to forget the phone numbers than the younger participants. So, if you're the kind of person who likes to talk on the phone while watching TV and cooking dinner, it may be harder as you grow older to remember what your phone conversation was about.

• *We don't process information as quickly*. Like other aspects of our functioning, the speed at which we process information can slow as we age. This may mean that we can't acquire something as quickly as we could previously. Also, we may not be able to absorb everything as well in a situation where we have a lot of information coming at us at once. Imagine yourself at a busy railroad station listening to the announcer quickly rattle off the train schedule. You will be able to learn and remember more of the schedule if you are in your twenties than if you are in your seventies. Are you doomed to miss your train if you are seventy-five? Of course not. It just means that you may not be "getting it" as quickly as you could before. Practice some simple techniques to manage how you process that information, though, and you will be able to *get* it, not *for*-get it.

• *We can't find the words to . . .* Are you suffering from "terminal word grope"? Many people begin to notice and complain about having a harder time finding that right word as they grow older. Although you may remember it at three o'clock in the morning, you may still be frustrated and even a little frightened. For some of us, these changes seem familiar. They certainly did for Letty Cottin Pogrebin, a well-known author and baby boomer, who wrote:

Of all the indignities of aging, involuntary malapropisms and memory lapses scare me most. I've always thought of words as power, the keystone of my "I may not be beautiful but at least I've got brains" self-image. I cannot conceive of who I'd be if my mind were to fail and the words got garbled for good.[3]

Scientists have attempted to explain this "tip of the tongue" phenomenon as a delay in levels of information processing. They suggest that while such experiences do increase in frequency with age, even older adults usually do recall the word or name eventually. And there are other factors we can work on that can make remembering words easier, as we shall see in Step 2.

## What Doesn't Change

Before these facts about memory and aging get you down, it's important to note how really minimal these changes are when you consider the overall complexity of our intellectual functioning. Long-term memory changes very little with aging. In addition, growing older has its rewards that come from being more experienced. For example, scientists have found that age has little impact on one's ability to perform at work. Often, older adults are better able to synthesize information and make sound judgments because of their past experience. As one leading aging expert observed, "While older adults probably do have deteriorating memory mechanisms that lead to increased memory failures, they probably also have enriched databases that enable them to perform some memory tasks more competently than younger adults, in spite of less effective memory systems."[4] Wisdom, after all, is something that we generally con-

[3] Letty Cottin Pogrebin, "Honey, What's Your Name Again?" *The New York Times,* 26 August 1996.
[4] M. Perlmutter, "An Apparent Paradox About Memory Aging," in *New Directions in Memory and Aging: Proceedings of the George A. Talland Memorial Conference,* edited by L. W. Poon, J. L. Fozard, L. S. Cermak et al. (Hillsdale, N.J.: Lawrence Erlbaum Associates, 1980), p. 353.

*Still Thinking After All Those Years*

Still worried that old age will bring you down? Consider these role models in healthy, productive aging:

| | |
|---|---|
| Grandma Moses | John Glenn |
| Benjamin Spock | Nelson Mandela |
| Tony Bennett | George Bush |
| Paul Newman | Brooke Astor |
| Strom Thurmond | Georgia O'Keeffe |
| Golda Meir | George Burns |

sider to come with age. So, instead of worrying about how much you forget, try marveling at how much you remember.

What, then, can we do about the changes in memory that come with aging? Quite a lot, actually. While we may not be able to reverse physiological changes that affect our ability to remember, we can practice healthy memory habits to strengthen our memory and help us get around these new challenges. Research has demonstrated again and again that we can improve our memory, even to the point of compensating for the losses that can be part of aging. Why, you could even remember *better* than you did at a younger age.

## Wake Up Your Memory with the A.M. Principle

While there is no easy trick or secret to making the most of your memory, there are simple steps you can take to improve how well you acquire and store information so you can remember it better. This book will help you learn these steps to maximize your memory fitness. How does the program work? Well, the backbone of this program can be summed up in the **A.M. Principle.** Here is a rule that, if you follow it, can help you *immediately* learn and remember more effectively. So let's wake up your memory with the A.M. Principle!

## A IS FOR ATTENTION

If you want to remember something, you have to pay attention to it. This may sound simple, but the most common reason healthy adults forget is because they fail to focus. Distractibility can account for memory lapses no matter what your age.

Here's an example:

> *I once had a call from Annie W., the mother of an acquaintance, who was in her late seventies and very concerned about how much she'd been forgetting of late. She wished to take my class, and enrolled for one scheduled to begin a few weeks later. When we spoke, I suggested that she try in the meantime to make an effort to really concentrate when she was learning something she wanted to recall later. The day before her class was to start Annie called. "Cynthia," she said, "I hope you won't mind, but I really don't think I need to come and take your course." I asked what had changed her mind. "Well," she responded, "I did what you told me and realized that I hadn't been paying any attention to the things I was so upset about forgetting. So I started to really try to pay attention and it worked. I'm hardly forgetting anything at all now."*

Attention is the most sensitive aspect of intellectual functioning. It is therefore quite vulnerable to being disrupted. In order to acquire information so we can later remember it, we must be mindful and focus on what we are trying to learn. In other words, the problem isn't that we forget, but that we don't "get" what we want to remember from the outset.

Does this sound easy to you? It is. But think for a moment of all the things in your daily life that you really don't pay attention to. Consider the following questions about information we encounter every day:

- *What color is at the bottom of the stoplight?*
- *What word appears over the image of George Washington on a quarter?*
- *What letters, if any, are missing from the telephone dial?*
- *How many light switches are in your house or apartment?*

How did you do? Chances are you don't know the correct answers to some of these questions, even though these are things that you come across, sometimes frequently, over the course of a typical day.[5] Why? Because we are not always mindful of things we do or see every day. But, you say, those are things I'm not *trying* to remember. Yes, this may be true. But I'll bet you're not really trying to remember where you put your keys down, either. Only by focusing our attention can we adequately acquire information and have it later when we need to remember it.

Can we improve our attention? Absolutely. How? Here are two basic habits we can develop to improve attention and maximize memory fitness immediately:

• ***Be aware.*** If you are aware that you are hearing or seeing something you want to remember, you will be more likely to pay attention to it, to "get" it, and to "have" it later when you want to

---

[5] The answers are: green; "Liberty"; Q and Z; and only you know!

remember it. Increased awareness of the need to remember will increase your attention toward that information.

Have you ever lost your car in a parking lot? Or forgotten whether you turned off the oven? Well, imagine if you had been more aware that you needed to be mindful of where you parked or whether you turned that knob. If only you had thought to yourself, "Okay, I need to pay attention now so I will remember what I'm doing." Being more aware in those situations would have encouraged you to pay closer attention and made it more likely that you would remember that information later.

• *Make the effort.* Next, you must try to focus your attention. As I tell my clients, being aware that you need to pay attention without making the effort to do so is like sleeping with the unread textbook under your pillow the night before final exams. It never worked, did it? Well, the same rule applies here. It isn't enough to know you must be mindful of something you want to remember: You must then do it. So when you park your car at the mall and want to be able to find it a few hours later, simply make the effort to look around and pay attention to where you are. Most likely there are some signs or other landmarks to help you remember where you've parked.

I still get a chuckle from this story:

*A family member of mine, at the time in his twenties, parked his car at an airport garage and left rather hurriedly to catch his flight. Upon his return several days later, he couldn't find his car. Quite upset, he reported it stolen to the parking lot attendant. The attendant, clearly a veteran of these circumstances, suggested that perhaps he had simply forgotten where he had parked. Being still young and rather confident of his memory, my relative insisted that his car had been taken, no question about it. The attendant finally convinced him to ride around in a cart to see if they could locate his car. Sure enough, they did . . . exactly where he had parked it. And was this young man embarrassed? You'd better believe it.*

We can promote our attention even further by identifying issues that may keep us from focusing clearly on things we want to remember. As we will see in Step 2, many factors in daily life can lower memory potential by making you more distracted and therefore less able to acquire information sufficiently. I see this with individuals who are especially busy (and who isn't these days?) or who may be more preoccupied than usual. A good example of this is Kathy L.:

*Kathy is a therapist in her early forties who was convinced that she was developing Alzheimer's disease. The memory lapses she was experiencing were particularly frightening because she had watched her mother suffer from that devastating illness beginning at a very early age. After a thorough evaluation and sev-*

---

### The Rainbow Casino

I recently heard about a casino where they painted each level of their parking garage a different color and then piped in music relating to each color on the appropriate floor. So, if you parked on the yellow level, you would hear "Tie a Yellow Ribbon Round the Ole Oak Tree." On the blue level, you might hear "Blue Suede Shoes." Seems like a pretty clever way to apply the A.M. Principle and help folks remember where they've parked!

*eral classes, Kathy realized that what was really getting in her way was her lifestyle: She was managing both an administrative position with a good deal of responsibility and a thriving private practice, maintaining two residences, and she had teenagers still at home. Kathy was able to recognize that her biggest obstacle to remembering was her distracted state of mind due to all the balls she was juggling. This realization alleviated a good deal of fear on her part and enabled her to work on ways to maximize her memory functioning.*

Often people who are worried about their memory are quite relieved when they realize that being distracted is the likely cause of their forgetfulness. Many of us can take some simple steps to get a better grip on things that are interfering with our attention, as we will see later.

---

## ■ HOT TIP ■
### *What Did I Come in Here For?*

Ever forget why you went into a room, or what it was you were going to do next? Does it make you feel like a memory flop? Relax—chances are you're distracted, so you lose your train of thought. Here's a tip: As you get up to go to the next room, repeat to yourself the reason you are going in there. For example, if you are going into the kitchen to find a pair of scissors, you can keep focused on that task by reminding yourself as you go: "I am getting the scissors, I am getting the scissors." While it might seem rather silly at first, it really works—and face it, it beats standing in the kitchen and muttering, "What was it that I came in here for?"

So, if you want to rev up your recall for something, you need to pay attention and make the effort to do so. You will *definitely* be better able to recall it later.

## M IS FOR MEANING

Material that is meaningful is memorable. The more meaningful something is to you, the more likely you are to pay attention to it and the easier it will be for you to learn. Giving meaning to information we want to remember also helps us control how that information is stored in our memory banks, making it more likely that we will recall it later. We tend to remember things that interest us for this very reason.

Much of what we would like to remember either has meaning or can be given meaning. Often we don't notice meaning that is inherent to something we wish to learn and recall. For example, a grocery list has an organization that, if used properly, can help us learn that list and give us a way to recall that information later. We can also impose meaning on information to make it more memorable. Techniques for making information easier to remember do not have to be complex or cumbersome. This program will introduce you to several simple memory habits you can adopt to help make information more meaningful and therefore easier to remember. Why, you even know some right now.

- How many days are in June? Did you say thirty? That's right, but how did you get there? If you recited to yourself, "Thirty days hath September, April, June . . . ," you just used a memory device to help you remember the correct answer.

- What do the following letters stand for: ASAP? Did you say "as soon as possible"? This is another example of a memory habit you already use. If you take a moment and think about all the acronyms you know and use, you'll see just how much you employ this particular technique.

Here are some other examples of how we can boost our brain-power by making information more meaningful:

• ***Organize it.*** Information that is organized is easier to learn and remember. Imagine you had a number of files that you used often. Would it be easier to find a particular file if you alphabetically organized them or if they were all just thrown in the file cabinet in no particular order? The answer is rather obvious. By imposing meaning—here, ordering the files according to an alphabetical scheme—you are able to more efficiently store and retrieve a particular file. Much of what we wish to remember either has an inherent organization or can have an organizational scheme imposed on it.

How we learn numbers is a good example of how we use organization to give information meaning. Try to learn the following numerical sequence:

7853420981

It will be easier to learn this number if you organize or "chunk" it into a few smaller groups of numbers. Since this number is ten digits long, you could chunk it like a phone number, a pattern that is meaningful to you as well:

(785) 342–0981

Organizing this string of numbers this way gives it meaning that will make it easier to remember. Many of us already use organization to help us remember.

• **See it.** We can also help give meaning to things we wish to remember by visualizing or seeing them. Try picturing in your head each item as you read the list below:

telephone
bird
bottle
square

Now look away and recall as many words on the list as you can. How did you do? Chances are that picturing this list of words helped you remember them. Why? Because for certain information we need to remember, our visual memory may actually be stronger than our verbal recall.

Seeing information is another way to give it meaning and make it more memorable. Think of all the things you need to recall that you can picture: Grocery items, phone numbers, e-mail addresses, and certain names are a few examples that come to mind. You can use your visual advantage to make information more memorable in a quick and easy way.

• **Connect it.** We can also make something we are trying to learn and remember more meaningful by connecting it with something we already know. Relating what you want to learn to something that is already familiar helps give it more meaning. Think of this as cross-referencing your brain. Examples include many spelling rules we learned in school. Can't remember how to spell the title of the person who runs your child's elementary school? Well, if you learned that "A princi*pal* is a prince of a *pal*," you'll have no trouble. This memory technique is a way of recalling how to properly spell "principal" by connecting the word with the spelling of a word you definitely know—"pal."

### The Overlearning Paradox:
### How to Improve Your Memory by
### Not *Paying Attention*

Do you waste a lot of time, not to mention aggravation, looking for things such as your keys, your glasses, or your wallet? One of the best ways to remember things we do often, such as putting down objects we use regularly, is by practicing a good memory habit so that we don't need to pay attention. This habit, called overlearning, is very simple and easy to do. By merely getting into the custom of always doing the same thing, we decrease our need to pay attention but are ensured that things will be predictable and consistent. A memory habit such as using a "forget-me-not" spot to keep track of your keys, glasses, and wallet is a great example of how you can use overlearning to your memory's advantage (see p. 113 in Step 4). Overlearning can be a very useful memory tool in many circumstances. Chances are you already use it and just need to learn how to apply it more effectively. After all, don't you have more important things to pay attention to?

Connecting information can also be a very powerful way to make it meaningful and memorable. Try the following: On a blank sheet of paper, draw an outline of Italy. Done? Great. Next, draw an outline of Peru. A little harder, perhaps? Can you guess why that may be the case? Well, chances are that at one time someone taught you to connect the outline of Italy with the shape of a boot. Yet no one taught you a similar technique for recalling the shape of Peru. That connection was a powerful tool you can still use, although elementary school may have been the last time you did so.

Later in the book we will learn more about these and other simple but impressive techniques to make information more meaningful and easier to remember.

Now that you are familiar with the A.M. Principle, you can begin practicing these basic techniques to apply attention and meaning to information you want to remember. You will instantly notice the difference once you've woken up your memory.

▪ STEP 1: QUIZ ▪

*Here is a brief quiz to help you see how well you paid attention to this step. Answer the following questions "true" or "false" (answers appear on page 36).*

**T  F**  1. If I try to hold someone's phone number in my memory temporarily until I can write it down, I am relying on my working memory.

**T  F**  2. If I train my memory, I will remember everything and forget nothing.

**T  F**  3. Most adults are too old to improve their memory.

**T  F**  4. The acquisition step of memory is relatively insensitive to distraction.

**T  F**  5. Paying better attention and giving meaning to information I need to remember will help me remember it more effectively.

**T  F**  6. Paying attention requires no special effort on my part.

**T  F**  7. "Long-term memory" is a term used to describe how we maintain information we want to keep over a greater period of time.

**T  F**  8. Visualizing information is not an effective means of improving my ability to recall it later.

**T  F**  9. Serious memory problems are an inevitable part of aging.

**T  F**  10. Practicing better memory habits will help me maximize my memory fitness.

■ STEP 1: ANSWERS ■

1. **True.** *Working memory is the process we use to hold a limited amount of information for a limited amount of time.*

2. **False.** *Forgetting is part of being human. Even individuals with trained memory forget from time to time. Practicing better memory habits will greatly improve your memory fitness, but will not give you perfect recall.*

3. **False.** *You are never too old to learn better memory habits and boost your brainpower.*

4. **False.** *The acquisition step of memory is very vulnerable to distraction. When we don't focus our attention on information we want to remember, we don't acquire it effectively. It's not that we forget it, but that we didn't "get" it to begin with.*

5. **True.** *Applying the A.M. Principle — attention and meaning — to something we want to recall later will maximize our memory potential.*

6. **False.** *Focusing our attention requires awareness and effort.*

7. **True.** *This question describes well the process of long-term memory.*

8. **False.** *"Seeing" something you wish to remember is an excellent way to make it more meaningful and therefore more memorable.*

9. **False.** *Serious memory problems are the result of disease. While you may be at greater risk for developing a memory disorder as you grow older, such problems are not necessarily part of the aging process. You may experience mild changes in memory function as you age, but*

such changes most likely will not get worse. You can improve your memory at any age by using better memory habits.

**10. True.** You can make the most of your memory by enhancing your memory health.

### ■ STEP 1: MEMORCISES ■

**1.** Who's playing games? You should be—games that involve sequencing or require you to work quickly are great for building up your attention span and information processing speed. Some terrific games include concentration, a form of solitaire that can be played with a simple deck of cards; Simon (Milton Bradley), an electronic game that is excellent for exercising your attention-span skills; word puzzles, brain teasers, and a myriad of computer games that require skill and speed. This week, look for games you enjoy playing that grab your attention and give it a real workout.

**2.** Write down a ten-digit number such as a phone number that you'd like to remember. Cover the number with a separate piece of paper so that only the first digit shows. Read that digit to yourself, then look away and repeat it. Add a digit each time you are successfully able to repeat the sequence. Once you have mastered the first number, use this technique to practice other numbers that you need to remember, such as credit card numbers and PIN numbers.

**3.** Go through the same steps as in Memorcise 2, only this time substitute randomly selected words instead of digits. Make sure that the words are unrelated and do not form a sentence. How many words can you hold in your short-term memory?

**4.** "Did You Notice?" games are games you can play anytime, anywhere for a quick attention-building fix. Here are some examples for you to try:

- After a social event, such as dinner with friends or a cocktail party, practice remembering details of the event with your spouse or a friend. Can you remember the names of people who were there, what people wore, the room's decor?

- Sit in your kitchen and make a list from memory of all the contents of your bedroom. Then do the same for all the contents of your medicine cabinet.

- On the bus or train, study the person opposite you for about a minute. Then look away, and review in your head all the details of his or her appearance to test how well you paid attention.

**5.** What do you do to exercise your brain? Think about what intellectual activities are part of your lifestyle that flex your brain "muscles." Do you read, solve crossword puzzles, play cards, paint, or take classes that interest you? Do you "cross train" your brain by doing things that challenge all the different aspects of your intellectual functioning? Do you need to do more?

# STEP
## 2

# The Lifestyle
# Connection

What has your day been like so far? How did you sleep last night? Did you exercise this morning? Did you eat breakfast? Take any medications? How was your commute? Was work stressful? Were you inundated with meetings, phone calls, and e-mail? Did you skip dinner so you could help your kids with their homework or catch up on work you'd brought home?

Why, you may be wondering, does this matter? Perhaps you don't see the connection between these issues and memory. In fact, many people who are concerned about their memory are unaware that the lifestyle choices they make from day to day affect how well they can remember. As you will see, there is overwhelming evidence that many aspects of our daily functioning influence memory performance. In fact, I have found that for many people such everyday life factors underlie the majority of their memory complaints. Often, when the question is "Why can't I remember?" the answer is: Look at your lifestyle.

Other memory programs rarely focus on the role of everyday life in memory function. In large part this is because their approach to memory improvement is to teach complex internal memory systems, not overall memory fitness. In addition, many of these "experts" are not health professionals and simply aren't aware of how important lifestyle is to memory. In this lesson, you will learn not only why the decisions we make about how we live matter, but how we can best deal with those factors in everyday life to maximize our memory power.

## How Daily Life Is Related to Memory

Why does how we live from day to day affect our memory performance? Very simply, memory is part of who we are. It does not exist in a protected "black box" in our heads; rather, memory is an integral aspect of our physical and mental functioning. Therefore, if we are not taking care of ourselves—for example, not getting adequate rest, or feeling very anxious—we may see an impact on our memory ability. Many people are unaware that their lifestyle choices matter until they become concerned about how well they are remembering. But when they realize how those choices affect memory, they are motivated to change them. Take the example of Trisha B.:

> *Trisha, a seventy-four-year-old retired social worker, was a self-described lifelong nervous wreck. At her group's last class, Trisha told me that our discussion about anxiety and memory made her realize how much her chronic anxiousness was getting in her way, not only when it came to remembering but in*

*all aspects of her life. As a result, she'd decided to finally do something about it, and had recently started a yoga class. She happily reported that she was feeling better—and more in control of her memory—than she had in years.*

How do these aspects of daily life affect our memory? In general, poor lifestyle choices compromise our memory potential by making it harder for us to focus our attention. Since attention is one of the most sensitive aspects of our intellectual functioning, it is quite vulnerable to influence from the ups and downs of everyday living. As we learned already, attention is central to memory, and we must be able to attend to information in order to acquire it. Factors in our lifestyle, therefore, can make it harder for us to focus on information and acquire it effectively.

Perhaps you can think of times when this has happened to you. You may occasionally have gotten tired and lost your train of thought. Maybe when you've been under a great deal of stress you were more forgetful. I am regularly regaled with stories about forgetting where lifestyle factors are the clear culprits. Here are some of my favorites:

*One Saturday a friend called me to go shopping. I was thrilled to go and was busy thinking about what I needed to buy. As I was about to walk out the door to meet her, I suddenly remembered that I was baby-sitting for my two-year-old granddaughter, who was asleep upstairs. Thank goodness I remembered in time!* —Arlene W., sixty-two-year-old medical researcher

*I was juggling a full-time job at a hospital in addition to a growing private practice at night. One day, I forgot an impor-*

*tant conference call at work. The next morning, my boss cut out an ad for a memory program and left it on my desk.*
—Kathy M., forty-seven-year-old education specialist

*After our second child was born, I was doing our grocery shopping when I drove away with the bags on top of the car. Luckily, someone stopped me before I'd gone too far.* —Mike B., thirty-nine-year-old attorney

Lest you think memory experts are immune, let me assure you that we are not. I have been known to forget what I was going to say or an errand I needed to run. And once, very distracted before starting a new class, I locked my keys in my office. The security officer in my building had a good chuckle about letting the memory teacher back into her office! At times like these, I know that life has caught up with me. No one can escape the effects of everyday life on their memory.

---

### Why This One's for You, Too

Sometimes people hear that I am speaking about lifestyle and memory and wonder whether it applies to them. "Sure," they think, "I can see why that's important . . . for someone else. But I'm young, I'm healthy, so it can't matter for me." The truth is, anyone who is concerned about their memory should be concerned about their lifestyle. Lifestyle factors account for a large number of the memory lapses that affect the healthy individuals I see. This is true especially for my younger clients. So listen up—this one's for you, too.

What can we do, then, to improve our memory fitness when it comes to our lifestyles? First, we can understand how the choices we make affect our ability to remember. From there, we can change how we cope with those factors to minimize their effects and make the most of our memory.

## Ten Lifestyle Factors Most Likely to Lower Your Memory Potential— and What to Do About Them

Good physical and emotional health are essential to promoting good memory fitness. Research has shown that the healthier we are overall, the healthier our memory will be. If we are not well, physically or mentally, it will often take a toll on our memory. Clearly, if you want to remember better, you need to take good care of yourself.

What does this mean, however? How can you maximize your memory fitness by taking good care of yourself? What lifestyle choices matter most? Let's look at the ten most common factors of everyday life that we know influence memory. As we review each one, we'll consider the bottom line: what we need to do to lessen its effect so we can make the most of our memory.

### 1  Physical Activity

We are all familiar with the importance of regular exercise to our physical health. Yet most of us don't appreciate how good physical activity is for the brain. Exercise is important to intellectual and memory health. Studies have demonstrated that exercise increases nerve growth factor in rats. This substance is essential to the function and survival of neurons, and it may protect neurons from free-radical damage (thought by many to underlie disease and aging).

Dr. Marilyn Albert and her colleagues found that adults are more likely to maintain sharp mental ability through aging if they are physically active and have good lung capacity, an indicator of cardiovascular fitness. Physical activity has also been associated with healthy aging.

How does exercise affect memory? Regular exercise improves the circulation of blood to your brain. This increase in cerebral blood flow gives your brain more oxygen and other nutrients the brain uses as "food." The result? You are more mentally alert and can learn and remember more effectively. Physical activity also helps your memory by lowering your risk for other diseases such as stroke, cardiovascular disease, stress, and depression, which can themselves affect memory ability.

**The bottom line:** If you want to improve your memory fitness, get to work on your physical fitness. Adding exercise to your lifestyle is a great way to improve your memory effectiveness, not to mention your overall well-being. And don't feel that starting an exercise program is a difficult hurdle to jump—something as simple as walking briskly for a half hour daily is great exercise and more than enough for starters. Many of my clients who begin a regular exercise program notice an almost immediate improvement in how well they remember. So just do it!

## 2 Diet

Maintaining a healthy diet is another very important way we can help ourselves remember more effectively. Experts have been telling us for years how we should be eating to avoid heart disease and other illnesses. Following a healthy diet also provides protection from the diseases that increase your risk for the second leading cause of memory disorder in this country: dementia resulting from stroke or other vascular diseases.

### Staying Memory-Healthy

I am often asked whether there is something we can do to keep our memory healthy as we grow older. Fortunately, there is growing evidence that we can largely determine how well we age based on how we live. And this includes how well our memory ages. Researchers with the MacArthur Foundation Consortium on Successful Aging followed a group of men and women in their eighties who had aged successfully and compared them with a similar group of individuals who had not fared as well (the results of this important study are chronicled in the book *Successful Aging* by Drs. John Rowe and Robert Kahn). These scientists looked specifically at the question of what distinguished successful agers from those older adults who had not remained mentally sharp. They found that subjects were more likely to have maintained mental ability through aging if they:

- *were physically active*
- *were better educated (which may be associated with greater mental activity)*
- *had good lung function (a rough indicator for cardiovascular fitness)*
- *had high self-efficacy, or a belief in their own ability to do well*

**The bottom line:** Eat a healthy, well-balanced diet that is low in fat. If you need to follow a special diet for health reasons, do it. We'll learn more about nutrition and memory in Step 3.

## 3 Mental Activity

How mentally active are you? Researchers have found that adults who report engaging in mentally stimulating activities are less likely to develop memory disorders and are more likely to age optimally. Mental stimulation appears to improve attention ability as well as intellectual processing speed and flexibility, which can slow with aging. We can increase our level of mental activity by getting into the habit of exercising our brains. The good news is that there are countless ways of getting a brain workout (see "Brain Games" box). Pursuits such as games, hobbies, and social gatherings are all ways we can give our brains a good dose of activity and boost our memory power.

***The bottom line:*** Think about how much mental activity you engage in on a regular basis. Adopt some ways of "exercising" your brain into your daily routine.

---

### Brain Games

Here are some ways you can work mental activity into your daily routine:

| | |
|---|---|
| Do crossword puzzles | Solve brain teasers |
| Play bridge | Read |
| Play board games | Play computer games |
| Do jigsaw puzzles | Paint |
| Do word-search puzzles | Take a pottery class |
| Play a musical instrument | Build a model airplane |
| Attend a class | Play card games |
| Join a reading group | Attend museum lectures |
| Learn a new language | Learn how to use a computer |

## 4 Medical Conditions

While many people are aware of the memory changes that occur with Alzheimer's disease or other dementias, most are unaware that even minor memory changes can be symptoms of other illnesses. An acute medical condition such as a viral or bacterial infection can temporarily lessen your ability to remember by making it harder

---

### *Medical Conditions That Can Affect Your Memory*

Many illnesses have been associated with changes in memory function. The list below is comprehensive but by no means exhaustive, and it does not include the progressive illnesses that primarily affect memory, known as the dementias. If you suffer from one of the conditions below and are concerned about your memory, you should speak with your doctor. Of course, you should speak with your doctor about any significant change in your memory function, even if you have not been diagnosed with another illness.

Cancer
Chronic fatigue syndrome
Chronic meningitis
Diabetes
Encephalitis
Endocrine imbalance
Folate (folic acid) deficiency
Hypertension
Infectious diseases
Lupus

Lyme disease
Multiple sclerosis
Normal pressure hydro-
cephalus
Parkinson's disease
Premenstrual syndrome
Thyroid imbalance
Toxic exposure
Vitamin $B_{12}$ deficiency

Source: C. R. Green and K. L. Davis, 1993.

for you to pay attention effectively. Older adults are particularly vulnerable to the temporary impact infections can have on memory. Chronic diseases such as diabetes, hypertension, Parkinson's disease, chronic fatigue syndrome, and multiple sclerosis have also been associated with memory problems. With many of these illnesses, memory changes are short-term and lessen as the underlying illness responds to treatment. However, some chronic conditions, such as hypertension and diabetes, have not only been associated with mild impairments in memory but can place individuals at greater risk for developing dementia.

If you have a medical condition and are concerned about being more forgetful than usual, discuss it with your doctor. He or she should be able to tell you whether those changes could be due to your illness.

Here's a story about the importance of managing your medical conditions.

*When I saw Matt J. for an evaluation, he was a fifty-four-year-old, highly accomplished top executive at a Fortune 500 company. Yet people around him were complaining that he wasn't himself. Matt couldn't seem to get anything done and would often forget conversations. When I met with Matt and his wife, I discovered that several years earlier he had been diagnosed with diabetes and hypertension. However, he had always been "too busy" to change his diet and lifestyle habits as his doctor suggested to control these illnesses, and he had had a hypertensive crisis that put him in the hospital for several days. Although he now makes more of an effort to follow his doctor's advice, my evaluation showed that damage had already been done. Matt had clear-cut intellectual impairments, most likely a result of his uncontrolled diabetes and hypertension.*

### *See, Hear, Remember*

A common medical condition that affects memory is sensory loss. We learn and remember things by seeing or hearing them. As we learned in Step 1, you cannot remember something you never learned in the first place. For that reason, you are at a serious disadvantage if you cannot effectively hear or see information you are trying to learn.

The best way to cope with losses in perceptual function is to use devices to counter those changes. By making the most of your vision and hearing, you will help yourself make the most of your memory. Yet the number of adults who need aids as the result of vision or hearing loss and don't use them or don't use them properly is surprising. A recent study found that few older adults with hearing loss actually use hearing aids, even if they're aware they need them. I have seen many individuals terrified that they were developing Alzheimer's disease who really weren't forgetting. They just weren't hearing what was being said.

What can you do? Get your vision and hearing checked regularly. If you need an assistive device such as glasses or a hearing aid, get them and use them. You have no chance of remembering what you aren't even seeing or hearing in the first place.

If you experience changes in vision and hearing that cannot be adequately addressed through assistive devices, try to obtain information you want to remember in ways that work best for you. Get large-print newspapers and books. Buy a tape recorder so you can listen again to presentations or TV shows. Use amplifying devices at theaters and on telephones. All of these aids will boost your chances of absorbing material that you want to remember later.

*The bottom line:* Be mindful of your body and its needs. Living a balanced lifestyle that includes a proper diet and regular exercise can lower your risk for developing certain medical conditions. If you are diagnosed with a chronic illness, following medical treatment in addition to a healthy lifestyle is essential. Several studies have shown that adequate long-term management of diseases such as diabetes and hypertension is important in warding off their potential impact on memory. Finally, if you are sick, take adequate time to recover. You are a person, not a machine. Providing yourself and your body with an opportunity to heal will help you recover more quickly and will decrease the likelihood of further complications from your illness.

### 5  Fatigue

Are you tired? Most adults in America are. Fatigue from sleep deprivation and overexertion is a common phenomenon in our culture. Why? Most likely because we simply do not give ourselves enough time to rest. Sleep researchers have suggested that we need more sleep than we typically get, certainly more than the gold standard of eight hours. In addition, our sleep may be disturbed, resulting in incomplete sleep cycles, which again can lead to fatigue. Finally, certain sleep disorders, such as snoring and breathing stoppage, have been associated with daytime sleepiness and lowered intellectual performance.

Getting enough sleep may be especially hard for older folks. Italian researchers found that 36 percent of the men and 54 percent of the women in a large community sample of older adults complained of sleep disturbance. Why is it harder to sleep when we grow older? First, physiological changes that are part of the aging process can increase urinary frequency in both men and women. As a result, older adults may wake more during the night

> ### Best Bets for a Good Night's Sleep
>
> Having trouble getting a good night's sleep? It happens to all of us at some time or another. Here are some tried-and-true tips to help you nod off and give your memory (and the rest of you) some much-needed slumber.
>
> - *Set up a regular bedtime routine.* Establishing good sleep habits is an important way you can help yourself sleep better. Such habits include having a regular bedtime, avoiding strenuous exercise in the evening, and practicing a relaxation routine prior to going to bed, such as deep breathing or taking a warm bath.
> - *Reserve your bed for sleep.* Many of us use our beds for sleep . . . and for reading, watching TV, talking on the phone, and paying bills. If you are having difficulty sleeping, save your bed for sleep only. Doing so will make it clear to your brain that this is the place for rest, not for the rent.
> - *Have a glass of warm milk.* Warm milk has often been used as a sleep aid. Milk contains tryptophan, a naturally occurring substance that induces relaxation.
> - *Use sleep medications sparingly.* There may be times when a sleep medication is the only thing that seems to help.

because they need to go to the bathroom. Also, older adults take more medications that may have the side effect of disrupting sleep. It's not that we need less sleep as we grow older, but rather that sleep is more difficult to get.

Why is fatigue so important to memory function? Fatigue directly interferes with attention. And you are well aware by now of what that means with regard to memory. Some studies have suggested that fatigue may also make it harder to recall information

While such agents are useful, particularly in acute cases of insomnia, their long-term use is not recommended. These medications are commonly benzodiazepines, which can as an unintended side effect lower memory performance. If you use a sleep medication, ask your doctor when the best time might be to consider stopping it. If you have difficulty sleeping without medication, you may wish to consult a psychologist who specializes in behavioral treatment of sleep disorders. Many of my clients report success with melatonin, a hormone supplement, and valerian, an herbal sleep remedy. However, scientific research on their efficacy is limited.

- *If sleep problems persist, talk to your doctor.* Insomnia and daytime drowsiness may be symptoms of something else. If the practical suggestions discussed above don't help you with your sleeplessness, talk to your physician about the difficulties you are having and what may be causing them. This is especially important if you are overweight and/or snore, both of which may place you at greater risk for sleep-related disorders.

stored in long-term memory. This may explain why at times it is harder to recall things we know well, such as words. Finally, fatigue is important because it is such a common complaint. In today's world we expect ourselves to achieve a lot. Doing it all is exhausting. And if something has to go to make time for all we need to do, it's usually sleep. Fatigue is an important influence on memory simply because so many of us live with it.

Fatigue is also a major factor in our ability to function effectively overall. It has been associated with impaired performance on tests of attention, problem solving, judgment, and memory, as well as with depressed mood and confusion. Human errors resulting in both minor and major disasters, from treatment mistakes in hospitals to the Chernobyl disaster, have been attributed to fatigue.

*The bottom line:* If you want to remember better, remember to get adequate rest. Practice proper sleep habits and leave yourself enough time to sleep so you feel rested upon awakening. If you have problems sleeping, try some of the simple, old-fashioned techniques in the box "Best Bets for a Good Night's Sleep." If you still have difficulty, talk with your doctor about what may be causing your sleep problems and how best to remedy them.

If you have a very active schedule, be certain to allow yourself breaks during the day. Take a breather, such as a walk around the block. It can also be helpful to alternate your activities between ones that require more effort and ones that are less demanding. Finally, if you can't get enough rest, don't be so hard on yourself. Sometimes we have little control over how much sleep we are getting. Realize that fatigue may be taking a toll on your memory. You can also compensate for the effects of fatigue by calling on your other memory fitness habits.

## 6 Medications

Medications are a hallmark of medicine, both ancient and modern. Substances ranging from herbs to powerful new pharmaceuticals developed using the latest technologies are available to treat a wide array of illnesses. Some treatments, however, have unintended side effects.

Memory is an area of functioning often vulnerable to the

unwanted side effects of medications. Several commonly used medications can lower our memory potential by interfering with attention. Substances such as antihistamines, antianxiety medications, and painkillers can hinder recall ability in this way. Certain recreational drugs, such as marijuana, also appear to inhibit new learning. Other medications, such as anticholinergic agents, disrupt memory by altering neurotransmitter function in the brain. Here's what happened to Myra R.:

*Myra R. came to see me several years ago for an evaluation. This fifty-three-year-old health scientist had noticed an increase in memory problems over the prior two years. Myra told me that she'd suffered from bad headaches for several years. Around the time of our meeting she'd been having a very hard time with them and was taking a number of medications, much more than she had in the past. When I reviewed these medications, I noticed that a number were painkillers that could interfere with memory performance. Myra's performance on a memory test indicated to me that her memory difficulties were most likely due to the medications she was taking. Myra discussed these findings with her doctor, who then worked with her to adjust her medications. As we expected, she found that simply changing her medications made a big difference to her memory function.*

Often doctors are not aware of the particular effects of a medication on memory. Sometimes research performed prior to a drug's approval may not include memory function, so that information is not available. A good example of this is oxybutynin chloride, an antispasmodic commonly prescribed to older adults for bladder incontinence. A study by Dr. Ira Katz and colleagues demonstrated

*Medications Known to Lower Memory Potential*

This list of medications that have been associated with changes in memory ability is not exhaustive, but it does include many of the more common substances that have been linked to memory changes. If you are worried about your memory, talk to your doctor about your concerns and ask if there is another treatment you could try. Many of us may not have a choice. If that is the case, we can still improve our memory by using good memory habits. **You should never stop taking a prescribed medication without discussing it with the doctor who prescribed it for you.**

- *Antihistamines.* Often used for treatment of allergies. Available over the counter.

- *Anticholinergics.* Previously used widely to treat depression. As the newer family of antidepressants, selective serotonin reuptake inhibitors (SSRIs), has become more popular, use of anticholinergic agents for depression has decreased. However, anticholinergics are used widely for treatment of other illnesses, such as bladder dysfunction.

- *Benzodiazepines.* Popular antianxiety medications. Also prescribed as sleep aids.

- *Beta-blockers.* Used for treatment of hypertension.

- *Opiates.* Frequently prescribed for pain management.

deficits in verbal memory and reaction time in a group of older subjects given this medication. Yet warnings regarding the adverse effects of this substance did not include information about its effects on memory performance.

We are especially vulnerable to the unintended side effects of medications when we grow older. Drug-related intellectual impairments are a common but preventable problem in older adults. As we age, our metabolism slows. As a result, a medication lasts longer in our bodies, placing us at greater risk for side effects such as memory difficulties. Those of us who specialize in memory disorders have seen cases of older adults suffering from delirium or cognitive impairment that turned out to be drug-related. Fortunately, drug-related memory impairments generally reverse once the culprit medication is discontinued. However, such confusion and impaired thinking may place older adults at increased risk for falls and other injuries. Proper care must be taken to adjust the medication dosage for older adults to guard against unwanted side effects.

Finally, medications may at times interact with each other to diminish our ability to recall information. Again, we are particularly susceptible to medication interactions as we grow older, since we tend to be prescribed more medications with increasing age, frequently by more than one physician.

What about medications to help memory function? There are currently no medications approved by the Food and Drug Administration for improving memory in healthy adults. However, research has demonstrated that certain substances may protect memory performance. One large epidemiological study found that subjects using nonsteroidal anti-inflammatory drugs (NSAIDs), such as ibuprofen, were less likely to develop Alzheimer's disease. However, NSAIDs are associated with other significant side effects, specifically gastrointestinal problems, which makes it difficult to recommend them for widespread use.

Research has also demonstrated that estrogen may play a role in maintaining good memory performance in older women. Findings on estrogen replacement and memory function are generally supportive, although the strength of such studies has recently been questioned (see "The Estrogen Equation" box). Finally, there are many popular herbal supplements reputed to improve memory performance. Unfortunately, the scientific evidence supporting their use is mixed. Many consumers are unaware that such supplements are indeed medications that may themselves have risks and side effects. We will focus more specifically on supplements commonly used as memory boosters in Step 3.

*The bottom line:* Be aware that the drugs you take can affect your memory, be they over-the-counter remedies, supplements, prescribed, or recreational drugs. Discuss with your doctor whether a medication you are taking is known to cause memory changes. **Please remember that you should never stop taking a medication without discussing it with the prescribing doctor.** Stopping a medication without first speaking with your physician may be dangerous, even life-threatening. If the medication you are prescribed is associated with increased memory problems, ask your doctor if other medications without such memory side effects might be available and appropriate. If no alternatives exist, your best bet is to build up other memory habits to help you compensate for any memory changes caused by medications.

If you are considering using an over-the-counter medication or supplement but are concerned that it may affect your memory performance, talk to a professional, such as your pharmacist or a nutritionist, who would be knowledgeable about that substance.

### 7 Depression

Have you ever felt depressed? Chances are you have, since a depressed mood is part of the normal range of human emotion. Feeling sad or blue is something we can all relate to. Think back to the last time you felt depressed. Did you have difficulty con-

### The Estrogen Equation

For several years scientists have been exploring the role estrogen plays in memory health as well as in overall cognitive function in women. Early findings suggested the hormone enhances new learning and helps women maintain verbal memory. Researchers also found evidence of a relationship between estrogen deficiency and Alzheimer's disease, a disorder that is more prevalent in women. As a result of this deeper understanding of estrogen's place in memory function, research next began to focus on the effects of estrogen replacement in healthy postmenopausal women. Several studies have generally found that maintained memory performance is a benefit of hormone replacement therapy. However, a few recent epidemiological studies have found no relationship between estrogen replacement and memory performance and no gender difference in the degree of memory loss associated with aging. Experts who study estrogen and memory are beginning to question the implications of these differing results and are calling for further studies of estrogen's role in memory function.

What's the bottom line in the estrogen equation? Use of hormone replacement therapy is a very personal decision that involves consideration of many risks and benefits. While further research is necessary before we can definitively conclude whether estrogen replacement can protect women from memory decline, any postmenopausal woman considering hormone replacement therapy should weigh the potential benefits for memory as well. Finally, women can supplement estrogen through diet, by eating foods high in phytoestrogen, such as soy-based products.

centrating? Was it harder to get things done? If your answer is yes, you'll understand how depression can affect memory.

When we are depressed, it is harder for us to pay attention and concentrate. In fact, being more distracted is one of the symptoms of a depressed mood. Why? Because we are preoccupied by whatever is upsetting us, be it a loss or a problem in our lives. As you know by now, paying attention is a crucial first step when we want to remember something. Since it's harder to do that when we're down, it will be harder to remember at those times as well.

Some of us may at times experience what experts call major depression. Major depression is an illness in which the feelings of depression or sadness become overwhelming and difficult to shake. The depressed mood can last for weeks or months and is often accompanied by feelings of listlessness, hopelessness, and anxiety. In many cases major depression interferes with the ability to function at work or at home. People suffering from major depression often complain of tremendous difficulty concentrating and, not surprisingly, of memory problems. Major depression is the most common mental illness and occurs with greater frequency in older adults. Approximately 6 percent of American adults over age sixty-five suffer from major depression. In fact, older adults will sometimes come to a doctor complaining of memory problems when depression is actually the root cause of their memory changes. In such cases, adequate treatment of the depression will result in improved memory performance.

*The bottom line:* When you are feeling down, don't worry about your memory. Keep in mind that when you are depressed you are likely to be preoccupied and less able to concentrate. You can help yourself remember better at those times by making sure to apply other good memory habits, such as getting organized and taking notes. What you don't need to do is worry about your memory, as it should improve once you are feeling better.

If your depressed feelings persist for several weeks or months and you are having a harder time managing your daily responsibilities at work or at home, please consider consulting a professional, such as your family doctor, a psychologist, or a psychiatrist. Major depression is a highly treatable illness and one that no person should have to live with.

## 8  Anxiety

We can all relate to feeling anxious from time to time. Perhaps you get nervous when making a presentation, or had butterflies in your stomach before your child's first day of kindergarten. Anxiety affects our memory ability in the same way it influences our performance in many other areas. The relationship between anxiety and performance can be illustrated by a graph that looks like an upside-down bell (see Figure 1). In order to perform effectively, we need to be primed or aroused. After all, if you're not concerned about how well you do something, you probably won't do very well at all. Arousal for performing a task improves your performance, up to a point of optimum balance between priming and task performance (this is the "top" of the upside-down bell). However, at some point we become too aroused or anxious. When that happens, anxiety interferes with our ability to perform the task, and performance declines. Why? When we are anxious we are (have you guessed by now?) more distractible. And we all know that being distracted makes it harder to remember.

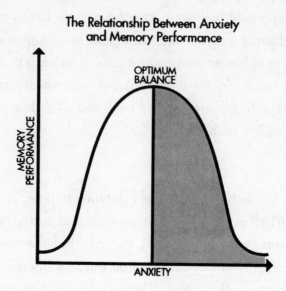

**The Relationship Between Anxiety and Memory Performance**

The balance between anxiety and performance varies from person to person and from task to task. In other words, what one person can do without breaking a sweat may lead someone else to run for cover. Finally, anxiety may make it harder to remember things that you know well, such as names and words. This may be one of the reasons why that word you can't recall all day comes to you in the wee hours of the morning, when you are less anxious about remembering it.

In some cases, feeling anxious pervades a person's life and becomes a mood they can't escape. Anxiety of such a degree can make it difficult for someone to function well at work or at home. Like major depression, anxiety disorders are highly treatable.

***The bottom line:*** Relax. If you get anxious about something you need to remember, you are only going to get in your own way. Try a quick "first aid" technique for calming down: Count backwards from twenty, take some deep breaths, stretch, or clear your mind. You will remember better if you are able to ease your anxiety.

If you find that you feel anxious a great deal of the time and that being anxious keeps you from doing things you need to for work or home, consider talking to a professional who specializes in anxiety disorders, who should be able to help you determine what kind of treatment will work best to reduce your anxiety.

### 9  Stress

Another lifestyle factor that can really zap your memory power is stress. Feeling stressed is, again, just another part of being human. But overwhelming stress can take a tremendous toll on our overall health, not to mention our memory.

How would you describe stress? For most of us stress is a feeling of pressure and lack of control. Yet formally defined, stress is merely the way you react to change. Stress in and of itself is not problematic. In fact, both "good" and "bad" life events are stressful. What distinguishes "good" stress from "bad" stress (distress) is the degree to which we feel we are in control. For example, most people would consider losing their job as more stressful than getting married. It is the sense of the former being more out of your control that makes it more distressful.

To understand how stress affects memory, let's look at what happens when we feel stress. When we experience stress, our body triggers a "stress adaptation" response, otherwise known as the "fight or flight" response. What happens?

- *Hormones, including adrenaline and glucocorticoids, are released*

- *Heart rate increases*

- *Breathing becomes more rapid and shallow*
- *Stored sugar is released by the liver*
- *Senses are heightened*
- *Muscles tense to prepare for movement*
- *Blood flow to digestive organs and extremities is restricted*
- *Blood flow to brain and major muscles increases*

This response to stress is a remnant of our primitive past. After all, this kind of preparation was essential if we were faced with something life-threatening, such as an attacking bear. Rarely today do we find ourselves in such life-or-death situations. But our bodies can't tell the difference between such events and the relatively mundane pressures of modern living, such as being stuck in traffic or getting into an argument with your spouse. The stress-adaptation response kicks in, again and again, exposing us regularly to low levels of this stressed condition.

This unrelenting chronic stress has been associated with various medical and emotional conditions, ranging from cardiovascular disease, gastrointestinal ailments, immune suppression, and endocrine changes. What about memory? Stress lowers memory performance secondarily because of its impact on overall health. Stress also makes us more distracted, which lowers our ability to acquire information we may want to remember.

There is growing evidence that stress may directly impair mem-

> *"A scattered mind cannot gather enough momentum*
> *to progress on the path to discipline."*
> — GURAMAYI CHIDVILARANANDA

ory function as well. Research has linked excess stress to shrinkage of the hippocampus, the area of the brain associated with new learning. Evidence for this has come from animal studies as well as studies in human populations exposed to excessive stress, such as individuals suffering from post-traumatic stress disorder. Scientists theorize that stress-induced increases of glucocorticoids are responsible for such changes. While more work is needed in this area, these findings suggest that stress is bad for memory in more ways than we previously understood.

---

### *Stress Busters*

Here are some great ways to minimize your stress and maximize your memory fitness:

- *Exercise.* Even walking for a half hour daily will give you a great stress break.

- *Start a hobby.* Activities such as reading, painting, playing games, or needlework all can help reduce stress.

- *Try the tried-and-true.* Specific activities for stress reduction have been around for centuries. Take a shot at yoga, tai chi, or meditation. Have a massage or try reflexology.

- *Pray.* Spiritual activities have long been a source of stress reduction. In addition to the personal release many experience with individual prayer, a spiritual community can give you support and solace.

- *Talk.* Being open and intimate with another person about your thoughts and feelings can help you balance your daily stresses.

*The bottom line:* Given these dire consequences, is there anything we can do about stress? The answer: Yes, lots. Research has demonstrated that balancing the ongoing stress in our lives through stress reduction habits can minimize the impact of stress on our health. What do these habits do? They simply shift focus away from what is stressful by moving our concentration to something else. Such habits don't have to be complicated. Activities such as exercise, hobbies, spiritual activities, or meditative activities are all stress busters (see "Stress Busters" box). Perhaps you already have a stress-balancing habit in your lifestyle. If so, that's great. If not, get one. Balancing stress is a great way to protect your memory, as well as your overall well-being.

## 10 Information Overload

Ever feel that you forget simply because you have too much to remember? I often hear this complaint, and I've used it myself. We have so much to remember: appointments, names, errands, PIN numbers, phone numbers, not to mention all those computer passwords. Also, we tend to fill many roles today, which increases the responsibilities we manage. Years ago a typical mother of two would have to remember tasks related to her family and home. Today that same woman may be working outside of the home, adding much more to what she needs to remember. I need only look at my own to-do list for this week to give you an example:

| DO | CALL |
|---|---|
| Write testing reports | Dr. Smith re: his patient |
| Do paper revisions | Dr. Rosell re: training |
| Organize boys' clothes | Baby-sitter for Saturday |
| Pick up dry cleaning | Melanie about car pool |
| Pick up photos | Painter |

My husband's list would also include tasks that a man of previous generations may not have had, such as carpooling and grocery shopping. More responsibility means more to remember.

Adding to the problem of how much we have to remember is the *pace* at which new information is presented to us. Technology has allowed us to receive information more quickly, which in turn has exposed us to greater volumes of information in the same time frame. The result? Information overload, or having too much to remember in too little time.

Why does information overload make it harder for us to remember? First, it is difficult to successfully focus our attention on a lot of material at once, which makes it less likely that we'll adequately absorb the information and remember it later. In addition, since our intellectual processing speed can slow as we age, it can be more difficult for us to learn things that come at us quickly. Our ability to acquire information is overloaded, and we simply can't "get" it all. And not getting it all can really become a problem. Take the following story from a client of mine:

*Jack F. is a forty-five-year-old self-employed engineer who came to see me because he felt he was having a much harder time remembering things at home and at work. He was most concerned about his difficulty recollecting conversations with his teenage son. It seemed that no matter what his son told him, Jack simply couldn't retain it. In our conversations, it became clear that Jack had trouble actually understanding much of what his son was saying, since his son would often speak very quickly and mumble (something many parents of teenagers can relate to!). It wasn't that Jack was forgetting what his son was saying, but rather that he wasn't "getting" it all, since it was coming at him too fast or too softly. Jack got in the habit of asking his son to slow down and speak up when they talked.*

*While at first his son was skeptical, Jack explained that he really wanted to know and remember the things his son was saying. Jack's persistence paid off. Once he was able to change the speed at which he and his son spoke, he became a more "memory-able" parent.*

**The bottom line:** Get control of information before it gets the best of you. Take charge of situations in which you are collecting information you want to remember. Take notes, ask people to slow down when they tell you something, space learning over time. Doing so will give you more opportunity to consolidate and learn the material you want to have later. Help yourself remember by using organizational techniques such as those described in Step 4. And don't be afraid to say, "I didn't get that, can you say it again?" Chances are the other person doesn't always get things the first time around, either.

So there are the ten lifestyle factors most likely to lower your memory potential. Of course there are other aspects of daily existence that can interfere with memory, but these are the most common culprits. You can get the most out of this lesson by doing the Memorcises to help you see how these factors may be lowering *your* memory power. Once you've identified which issues are getting in your way, you can begin to do something about them. Coping effectively with these lifestyle factors will help you move forward on the road to better memory fitness.

### How Much Is More?

Often people will tell me that they are more forgetful than their parents and grandparents were because they have more they need to remember. While we have a great deal of information coming our way, I often wonder if previous generations didn't have *more* to remember than we do today. After all, they didn't always have the benefit of buying prepared foods and off-the-rack clothing. I was recently reading *Little House in the Big Woods* by Laura Ingalls Wilder to my children, and I came across the following passage, which shows how much our forebears had to keep in mind:

Pa skinned the deer carefully and salted and stretched the hides, for he would make soft leather of them. Then he cut up the meat, and sprinkled salt over the pieces as he laid them on a board.

Standing on end in the yard was a tall length cut from the trunk of a big hollow tree. Pa had driven nails inside as far as he could reach from each end. Then he stood it up, put a little roof over the top, and cut a little door on one side near the bottom. On the piece that he cut out he fastened leather hinges; then he fitted it into place, and that was the little door, with the bark still on it.

After the deer meat had been salted several days, Pa cut a hole near the end of each piece and put a string through it. Laura watched him do this, and then she watched him hang the meat on the nails in the hollow log.

He reached up through the little door and hung meat

on the nails, as far up as he could reach. Then he put a ladder against the log, climbed up to the top, moved the roof to one side, and reached down inside to hang meat on those nails.[6]

[6] L. I. Wilder, *Little House in the Big Woods* (New York: Harper Trophy, 1932), pp. 6–7.

■ STEP 2: QUIZ ■

*This quiz will help you know if you got the most out of this lesson. Answer the following questions "true" or "false" (answers appear on page 72).*

**T  F**   1. I have little control over how tired I am.

**T  F**   2. Many factors in my daily life affect my memory by making it harder for me to focus my attention.

**T  F**   3. Physical exercise will not help my memory.

**T  F**   4. Fatigue can lower my ability to learn new information, but has no impact on how well I can recall information I knew previously.

**T  F**   5. Estrogen plays no role in memory function in women.

**T  F**   6. If I am overly anxious when learning something, relaxing will improve how well I can learn it.

**T  F**   7. Information overload can be defined as having to carry around too large an appointment book.

**T  F**   8. My emotional state has no effect on my memory.

**T  F**   9. The goal of stress management is to help us avoid stress.

**T  F**  10. Stress affects memory indirectly by its significant impact on our physical and emotional health.

■ STEP 2: ANSWERS ■

1. **False.** *While at times it may feel as if you have little control over how tired you are, chances are that you could be less tired if you practiced better sleep habits, gave yourself opportunities to rest, and planned ahead so you could better balance your schedule between demanding activities and those that are less strenuous.*

2. **True.** *Many of the factors discussed in this lesson affect memory fitness by making it harder to focus your attention effectively on information you are learning, so that you are less likely to acquire it.*

3. **False.** *Physical exercise is important to your overall well-being and therefore is important to your memory functioning as well. In addition, physical exercise may help memory and other intellectual functions by improving the circulation of blood to your brain.*

4. **False.** *Researchers have found that fatigue impacts our ability to recall well learned information in addition to interfering with new learning.*

5. **False.** *Several studies have suggested that postmenopausal women receiving hormone replacement therapy fared better with regard to memory performance than those who were not. These findings suggest that estrogen plays a meaningful role in memory function for women.*

6. **True.** *If you are anxious when you are trying to learn new information, chances are that your anxiety will interfere with your ability to absorb that information effectively. Relaxing will allow you to focus on the task at hand, putting you in a better position to learn and remember the information.*

**7. False.** *Information overload refers to situations where we are faced with learning too much information too quickly. If you're concerned about carrying around too large an appointment book, don't worry — we'll get to that in Step 4.*

**8. False.** *Emotional distress, most specifically anxiety and depression, can make it harder for us to learn and remember information, since we are likely to be more distractible when we are upset.*

**9. False.** *The goal of stress management is to help us cope with stress more effectively. We cannot avoid stress altogether — it is part of the human experience. Nor should we want to avoid stress, since many happy events, such as getting married or getting a promotion, are stressful but worth it!*

**10. True.** *Stress affects memory through its impact on our physical and emotional health, which in turn can lower our memory potential.*

## ■ STEP 2: MEMORCISES ■

1. Identify a specific activity in the coming week that will require your memory to be at its best. Next, consider which of the ten lifestyle factors discussed may interfere with your ability to achieve your memory potential at that time. Then consider what you can do to cope more effectively with those factors to minimize their impact and maximize your performance.

Activity: _____

_____

_____

_____

| *Lifestyle factors that may interfere with my memory effectiveness:* | *Coping skills I can use in dealing with these lifestyle factors:* |
|---|---|
| 1._____ | _____ |
| 2._____ | _____ |
| 3._____ | _____ |
| 4._____ | _____ |
| 5._____ | _____ |
| 6._____ | _____ |

2. Which of the lifestyle factors from Step 2 matter most to you? Figure out which issues are lowering your memory potential the most. Then commit yourself to developing better habits for dealing with them to help make the most of your memory.

*Lifestyle factor:*                    *How I will deal with it:*

1. _____    _____

2. _____    _____

3. _____    _____

4. _____    _____

5. _____    _____

6. _____    _____

# STEP
## 3

# Food for Thoughts

---

■ **IN THIS STEP YOU WILL LEARN:** ■

*How Diet Is Related to Memory*
*The Best Diet to Boost Your Brainpower*
*Plus the Scoop on Supplements*

---

Are you familiar with the expression "You are what you eat"? Chances are you've heard this phrase before. But have you ever really thought about what it means? Most of us know that nutrition influences our overall health. Yet we still seem to have difficulty making the connection between what we eat and how well our bodies function day to day. In the same way that diet plays an important role in our overall well-being, diet influences memory. In this lesson, we will give some thought to food and how what we eat can help us maximize our memory fitness.

## How Diet Is Related to Memory

What is the connection between what you eat and drink and how well you can remember? Let's look first at why diet is important to our memory's functioning.

• ***Diet is an important factor in our overall health.*** It is a widely accepted fact that what we eat affects our well-being. Through our diet our bodies get the nutrients they need to function. Science has demonstrated again and again how important healthy eating is to living well. Conversely, we know that inadequate nutrition can lead to neurological and other health problems. Also, what we eat may make us more vulnerable to certain diseases.

As we learned in Step 2, memory is part of our overall health picture. Therefore, anything that affects our total fitness will impact our memory health as well. Nutrition is an important concern for memory because it affects our overall well-being.

• ***Diet plays an important role specifically in memory health.*** A healthy memory requires fit brain function. The energy that the brain needs to work comes, of course, from the nutrition provided by diet. In this way nutrition directly influences memory fitness. Our diet gives us the energy we need to remember.

The other side of the coin, of course, is that what we eat can *adversely* affect our memory function. Certain unhealthy diet patterns can make it harder to remember. I sometimes see patients with changes in memory function because of such behaviors. For example, I once evaluated a woman in her twenties who had been hospitalized for an eating disorder; her doctors were concerned that she appeared confused at times and was having difficulty following directions. I found that she was suffering from subtle but clear changes in her intellectual functioning, including the area of verbal memory. Further studies found atrophy, or shrinkage, of certain areas of her brain. These changes were most likely due to the maladaptive dietary patterns that were part of her illness. Finally, certain diseases that can specifically affect memory, such as hypertension and diabetes, can be influenced by what we eat.

What and how we eat plays an important role in reaching maximum memory potential.

## The Best Diet to Boost Your Brainpower

How, then, can we eat to remember? Is there a specific diet we should follow? A particular supplement to stock up on? A sound diet for memory doesn't have to be complicated. And you're more likely to stick to a nutritional plan you can really follow. Here are some simple tips on how you can help yourself get the best food for thoughts.

### 1 Eat a healthy, well-balanced diet.

One of the most important things you can do for your memory is simply to eat well. Brain cells—indeed, all body cells—need adequate nutrition for normal activity. Current dietary guidelines suggest that a varied diet that is low in fat and high in fruits, whole grains, vegetables, and protein is best. Fruits and vegetables can also be important food sources of antioxidants, food components that may provide protection from disease and aging. The U.S. Department of Agriculture's recommended dietary guidelines are a great resource for figuring out exactly what a well-balanced diet should include (see box, "What Is a Well-Balanced Diet?").

### 2 Eat often.

You can benefit more fully from your diet if you spread your nutritional intake evenly over the course of the day. Rather than eating three large meals, try planning six smaller meals during your day. If that's too cumbersome, aim for three medium-sized meals with three snacks in between. Your body will absorb nutrients more efficiently, allowing you to get the most from your food.

### *What Is a Well-Balanced Diet?*

While we've all heard the term "well-balanced diet," many of us are unsure exactly what it means. Here are the recommended guidelines from the U.S. Department of Agriculture. Use it to help figure out what you should be eating:

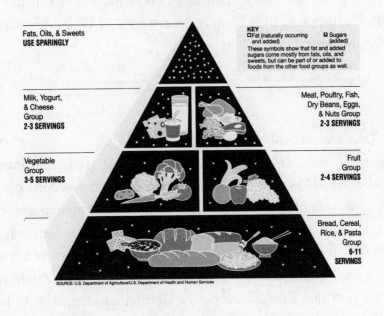

**Food Guide Pyramid**
A Guide to Daily Food Choices

Fats, Oils, & Sweets
USE SPARINGLY

KEY
☐ Fat (naturally occurring     ▨ Sugars
and added)                          (added)
These symbols show that fat and added sugars come mostly from fats, oils, and sweets, but can be part of or added to foods from the other food groups as well.

Milk, Yogurt,
& Cheese
Group
2-3 SERVINGS

Meat, Poultry, Fish,
Dry Beans, Eggs,
& Nuts Group
2-3 SERVINGS

Vegetable
Group
3-5 SERVINGS

Fruit
Group
2-4 SERVINGS

Bread, Cereal,
Rice, & Pasta
Group
6-11
SERVINGS

SOURCE: U.S. Department of Agriculture/U.S. Department of Health and Human Services

**3** **Drink often.**

We frequently forget the importance of liquids in our diet. Yet adequate hydration is important to all our body tissues, including our brains. Drinking approximately thirty-six to sixty-four ounces of water daily will help keep those thoughts flowing.

■ HOT TIP ■
*What's New in Nutrition*

Need a reliable resource for nutritional information? The
Center for Science in the Public Interest, a nonprofit health-
advocacy group, publishes the *Nutrition Action Healthletter.*
The Center also conducts independent research on our
favorite foods (such as movie-house popcorn) and supple-
ments. You can reach them at: Center for Science in the
Public Interest, 1875 Connecticut Avenue N.W., Suite 300,
Washington, D.C. 20009.

4 **Take a good multivitamin.**
In general, your daily food intake should meet your major nutritional needs. However, there may be times when you don't eat as
well as you should, or your diet may not routinely include sources
for certain essential vitamins or minerals. What's the best way to
be sure that your brain is getting all it needs to remember better?
Add a good multivitamin to your daily routine. A multivitamin is a
terrific nutritional insurance policy. Getting into the habit of taking one can guarantee you get adequate amounts of important substances you might otherwise miss. Look for a multivitamin that
contains a wide range of essential vitamins and minerals. The best
multivitamin for memory should include 100 percent of the recommended daily allowance (RDA) of vitamins $B_6$, $B_{12}$, and folic
acid (folate) in addition to the minerals zinc and boron. The good
news is that most multivitamins from reputable sources already
contain adequate levels of these substances.

## ■ HOT TIP ■
### *Maxing Out on Your Multi*

Want to get the most out of your multivitamin? Get into the habit of taking your multivitamin at lunch. Your body will absorb the nutrients in a multivitamin better when it's taken in the middle of the day and at a meal, when you are already digesting. Also, look for a multivitamin in liquid or powder form, both of which are more easily absorbed than hard tablets.

---

**5** **Add some antioxidants.**

One of the most prevalent theories of aging is the free-radical theory. "Free radicals" are by-products of normal oxygen metabolism in the body. According to this theory, free radicals wreak havoc on other cells, causing damage that results in disease and aging. Antioxidants are substances that absorb free radicals, thereby protecting us from the harm they do.

While much antioxidant research has taken place in other areas of aging and disease, experts are beginning to find that antioxidants are important in protecting memory function as well. Researcher W. J. Perrig and colleagues looked at the relationship between antioxidants and memory performance in a group of 442 healthy older adults. The analyses they performed focused on this relationship both immediately and over an eighteen-year period. The researchers found that higher levels of antioxidants in the blood were associated with better memory performance. Other researchers found that vitamin E, considered by many to be one of the most powerful antioxidants, slowed the progression of Alzheimer's disease.

*Eating for Antioxidants*

You don't need to pop another pill to get your daily dose of antioxidants. The foods below are high in antioxidants—and good for you as well:

| | |
|---|---|
| Beets | Plums |
| Blueberries | Potatoes |
| Broccoli | Red grapes |
| Corn | Red peppers |
| Kale | Spinach |
| Kiwi | Strawberries |
| Oranges | Sweet potatoes |
| Pink grapefruit | White grapefruit |

Source: *Nutrition Action Healthletter,* May 1997.

Given this evidence, it's a good idea to add an antioxidant to your diet. While your multivitamin probably includes several antioxidants, you can supplement your diet further by adding an additional dose of vitamin C, vitamin E, or beta-carotene to your vitamin intake. You can also increase your antioxidant dose through your diet (see "Eating for Antioxidants" box). Again, add only moderate amounts of these antioxidants to your diet. While the risks from taking too much of any of these supplements are relatively minimal, overdosing on them is not a good idea.

**6** **Take care with caffeine.**

Have you had some caffeine today? If so, you are not alone. Caffeine is ever present in the modern diet. While many of us associate caffeine with coffee, it is also found in black and green teas and caffeinated soft drinks, as well as chocolate.

As you may know, caffeine is a drug, a stimulant that heightens our awareness and ability to respond. In fact, at low doses, caffeine can be helpful to memory. By aiding attention, caffeine can improve our focus and make it easier for us to learn and remember. It is for this reason that I often joke to my students that caffeine is our drug of choice for dealing with fatigue. At higher doses, however, caffeine can be overstimulating and interfere with attention and concentration, making it harder to remember.

When does caffeine go from being just enough to becoming a problem? That depends on the individual. Many factors, such as weight, gender, and age influence how you tolerate caffeine. When it comes to how caffeine affects your memory, you are your own best judge. Drinking some caffeine may be helpful. However, you are more likely to have difficulty remembering when you use caffeine to the point of feeling jittery or distracted. The best way to use caffeine is to strike a balance for yourself. Just keep in mind that when it comes to caffeine and memory, less is more.

**7  Be wary of the sugar bowl.**
Sugar is another substance common in our diet that can affect our memory performance. Our brains use energy in the form of glucose, or simple sugar. Could a little sweetness therefore help move our memory along? The evidence is mixed. Some scientists have found that small amounts of sugar intake can temporarily enhance learning. This is particularly true for older adults, who may experience some minor alterations in glucose regulation. Yet other researchers have found that a diet high in sugar interferes with memory functioning in the long run.

What strategy should you use to handle sugar in your diet? Again, your best bet is to be aware of your sugar intake. If you want to experiment with the impact sugar has on your memory, try having a high-sugar snack, such as jelly beans or a sugared soft drink, and notice for yourself its effect on your thinking. Are you stimulated or jittery? Are you focused or flighty? Also, if you tend to "crash" after a high-sugar snack, make sure to avoid such foods prior to an event where you need your memory to be at its best.

Here's one of my favorite stories about how changing your diet can make it easier to remember:

*Jay W. came to my class several years ago. A forty-three-year-old locksmith with a thriving business, Jay was finding it increasingly difficult to keep in mind all the details he needed to remember. When we reviewed the relationship between sugar and memory function in class, Jay looked as if a light-bulb had just gone on in his head. In his travels from job to job, Jay would often indulge in a little "pick-me-up" snack— a doughnut in the morning, a candy bar in the afternoon. And when he thought about it, he did feel more out of it after those little treats. After a few weeks of experimenting with healthy snacks such as fruit and nuts (and, let's face it, gaining willpower), Jay happily reported a noticeable improvement in his memory.*

## 8  Be alert to alcohol.

Another common substance in our diet is alcohol. Like caffeine, alcohol is a drug. As a depressant, alcohol inhibits normal neuronal activity. The result? Alcohol may help you feel more relaxed and calm. However, it won't help you remember any better. In fact, there is ample scientific evidence showing that alcohol, even in small amounts, interferes with new learning. Heavy use of alcohol within a short span of time can result in memory loss for the period of intoxication, sometimes referred to as an alcoholic blackout. Significant long-term use of alcohol, such as that seen in alcohol dependence, has been associated with a form of memory disorder known as alcohol-related dementia.

Does all this mean you shouldn't drink any alcohol? Of course not. Moderate use of alcohol, such as a glass of wine with dinner, can be enjoyable and may have other beneficial health effects. Bear in mind, however, that alcohol can interfere with your memory ability for the time you are drinking. Balancing your alcohol intake accordingly will allow you to manage its impact on your memory. Only you know how much alcohol is enough. Finally, if you drink heavily, be aware that you may be placing yourself at risk for memory problems (in addition to other serious illnesses). There are many good reasons to take control of your drinking, and ample resources to help you do it.

### 9  Be skeptical about supplements.

These days it seems like everyone has a special tonic for memory lapses. Ginkgo biloba, choline, DHEA, phosphatidylserine, L-carnitine, vinpocetine—these are just a few of the "memory cures" I've been asked about. Herbal and other natural remedies have become so popular that the nutritional supplement business has become a multibillion-dollar industry. Unfortunately, it is an unregulated industry that does not need to meet Food and Drug Administration standards and is not overseen by any government agency. Nutritional supplement companies therefore have wide discretion in the claims they make about their products. In other words, you have no way of knowing whether such claims are backed by scientific evidence. You don't even have a guarantee that what they claim is in their product is actually there.

I advise my clients to be savvy about supplements. It may be tempting to think that a pill from all-natural sources can magically improve your memory. However, there are several reasons to be a cynic when it comes to supplements:

- *You don't need a "memory cure."* As I've said before, why would you need a cure for something that isn't broken? For most adults, remembering better is simply a matter of better memory fitness. The best cure for your memory is already within your control. Gallons of "memory tonic" won't help you if you aren't making good memory habits part of your life.

- *The proof that supplements really work is mixed.* While it is possible that some supplements may help, many claims of their effectiveness simply aren't proven. Until there is better oversight of the supplements industry, you should be wary of the benefits advertised by the companies selling them. Often the scientific evidence is more mixed than they would lead you to believe.

- *Natural isn't necessarily better.* Many folks have been misled into thinking that because something is natural or from a different healing tradition it is safe and better than what modern medicine has to offer. Make no mistake: Supplements—herbal, natural, alternative—are drugs. In fact, many of the substances we consider traditional drugs, such as aspirin and penicillin, are natural. Just because a drug is herbal doesn't mean it's safe to take. People have experienced side effects, some quite serious, from taking herbal supplements. Surely you would think twice about taking a powerful cardiac medication just because you could buy it at the grocery store. Also, there have been reports of individuals having dangerous reactions to certain supplements, often when the supplement was inadvertently contaminated during processing. Hopefully, future regulation of the supplements industry, either voluntary or imposed, will minimize the risk of such events for individuals using supplements.

Does this mean you shouldn't try any supplement for your memory? Not necessarily. You may want to experiment with these substances to see if you find them helpful. You'll find the latest information about the most popular memory supplements in the box "Should You Give It a Ginkgo? The Scoop on Supplements." If you want to try a supplement, make sure you get it from a reputable company. You should discuss using a supplement with your doctor first, especially if you have a chronic medical condition or are on any medications. (There could be potentially dangerous drug/supplement interactions.) While your doctor may not know much about a particular supplement, try to provide him or her with as much material as you can about it so that he or she can help you make an informed decision. Look for information about different supplements at the library or in objective sources, such as university health newsletters.

---

### Can What You Eat Cause You to Forget?

Memory loss can be a symptom of many conditions, including food poisoning. A 1997 outbreak of the toxic microbe *Pfiesteria piscicia* in the Chesapeake Bay area caused serious cognitive impairment, including memory loss, in dozens of people exposed to the infected water. While they are rare, such cases do occur.

## Should You Give It a Ginkgo?
## The Scoop on Supplements

Whether or not to take a "memory booster" is on a lot of people's minds. To help you decide, here's the latest scientific information on the most popular herbal supplements for memory:

### Ginkgo Biloba

Ginkgo biloba, also known simply as ginkgo, is an extract from the leaves of the *Ginkgo biloba* tree. Used in Chinese medicine as a treatment for circulatory disorders and memory disturbances, this drug dilates the blood vessels, allowing improved circulation. Ginkgo is one of the most popular supplements for memory, especially in Germany. But is it effective? The majority of studies on ginkgo have looked at its usefulness in treating dementia. The results of these studies have been mixed. As a result, ginkgo has not received wide support in the scientific community. Also, there is little evidence that ginkgo improves memory function in *healthy* adults. Ginkgo may be harmful to anyone on prescription medication or with a blood-clotting disorder. While theoretically ginkgo could help you remember better by getting more blood to your brain, you can achieve that just as effectively by exercising regularly. But if you want to try an herbal memory remedy, this is the one that has been most widely studied and has a long tradition of use in Eastern medicine.

### Choline

Choline is an essential part of the cholinergic neurotransmitter system, which plays an important role in memory function.

It is found in many common foods, such as soybeans, peanuts, and egg yolks. There is no clear evidence that supplementing your diet with choline can improve memory function. Enough choline, however, will make you smell like a fish (probably not the effect you are looking for).

## Phosphatidylserine (PS)

This phospholipid has recently received attention as a memory booster. Studies in persons with mild memory impairment have suggested that PS may be helpful, although probably not to the miraculous extent its advocates claim. Also, the majority of studies used a form of PS derived from cows' brains, which was withdrawn from production following the "mad cow disease" scare several years ago. A soy-derived form of PS is now available, but its effectiveness is even less certain.

## DHEA

DHEA, a natural precursor to estrogen and testosterone, has been touted not only as a supplement to boost memory but also as a cure for anything that ails the aging body. DHEA levels do decrease with age, and low DHEA has been associated with illnesses such as diabetes, osteoporosis, and dementia. However, there is little evidence that the claims made on DHEA's behalf are true. More seriously, DHEA may have significant negative health effects, such as liver damage and heart palpitations, and may encourage the growth of prostate cancer. Until further testing is done, your best bet with DHEA is to avoid taking it.

In sum, eating to remember is another way we can work better memory fitness into our lives. Follow the nine simple suggestions in this step to give your memory the nutritional advantage it needs to be at its best. As I said earlier, eating better for brainpower doesn't need to be complicated. In many ways, these guidelines are similar to any geared to improving overall health. By incorporating them into your lifestyle you'll give yourself the most food for thoughts.

■ STEP 3: QUIZ ■

*Here is a quiz to get your brain working. Answer the following questions "true" or "false" (answers appear on page 92).*

**T  F**  1. What I eat has no impact on how well I remember.

**T  F**  2. Having a couple of beers may make it harder to remember a phone number given to me by someone I've just met.

**T  F**  3. Even a little caffeine is bad for memory.

**T  F**  4. Eating several smaller meals over the course of the day instead of three large ones will help me remember better.

**T  F**  5. Herbal supplements are a proven way to improve my memory effectiveness.

**T  F**  6. Water is a good source of antioxidants.

**T  F**  7. Taking a multivitamin is a way to get the nutrients I need every day.

**T  F**  8. A high-sugar diet will help me remember better.

**T  F**  9. A healthy diet may protect me from certain chronic diseases associated with memory loss.

**T  F** 10. Eating well is just one of the many ways I can maximize my memory fitness.

■ STEP 3: ANSWERS ■

**1. False.** *Taking good care of yourself by eating a well-balanced, healthy diet is important to your overall memory fitness.*

**2. True.** *Studies have shown that alcohol inhibits our ability to learn new information at the time that we are drinking.*

**3. False.** *A little caffeine can boost attention and concentration, which will make it easier to retain things you want to remember. Too much caffeine, however, can have just the opposite effect. The key to caffeine is balance.*

**4. True.** *Providing your brain with consistent doses of nourishment throughout the day is a practical way to make the most of your memory.*

**5. False.** *Findings on herbal supplements are mixed, and no one supplement has been proven to improve memory function.*

**6. False.** *Water is good for you, but it does not contain antioxidants.*

**7. True.** *A daily multivitamin is a great insurance policy that you are getting what you need in your diet.*

**8. False.** *While a high-sugar snack immediately before a demanding memory task may help some people, this is not true for everyone. In addition, there is no evidence that a diet consistently high in sugar is good for your memory. In fact, such a diet may place you at greater risk for certain chronic diseases that can lead to memory impairment.*

**9. True.** *Eating a well-balanced, low-fat diet may provide protection from conditions such as diabetes and hypertension that can impact memory.*

**10. True.** *Following a diet that is good for your memory is one wonderful way to improve your memory fitness.*

■ STEP 3: MEMORCISES ■

1. Over the next week, become more aware of your diet. How many of the tips outlined in Step 3 do you already follow? Which do you need to work on?

2. Keep track of the impact sugar has on your memory and on your overall functioning. Notice what happens after you have a sugary snack. Is it harder for you to think clearly? Do you experience a "sugar slump"? If you're not sure, try this test: Avoid sweets for approximately eight hours. Then, eat a sugary snack, such as a sugared soft drink or jelly beans. Note your reaction. Remember how sugar affects you the next time you are tempted to indulge yet need your memory to be at its best.

3. Keep an eye on the java. Over the next week, keep track of how much caffeine you drink or eat. Remember that caffeine can come not only from coffee, but also from tea, caffeinated soft drinks, and chocolate. Notice where your threshold is between when caffeine helps you feel stimulated and when it makes you jittery.

4. If you don't already take a multivitamin, consider adding one to your diet. Go to your local drugstore and research which multivitamin will work best for you. Make sure you look for one that has folic acid (folate), $B_6$, $B_{12}$, zinc, and boron. Consider taking a liquid or powder form of multivitamin, both of which are becoming more widely available.

# STEP
4

# Get Organized

■ **IN THIS STEP YOU WILL LEARN:** ■

*Why We Need Memory Tools*
*The Best Tools for Remembering What You Need to Do*
*The Best Habits for Remembering What You Need to Do*
*How to Remember What Was Said*
*How to Remember Where Things Are*
*More Great Memory Tools*
*Ten Top Tips for Getting Organized*

How much do you have to remember? If you're like most people I know, chances are quite a lot. Meetings for work, presents to buy, doctors' appointments, where you put your tickets for that concert next week, the snacks you promised to bring to your daughter's next soccer game . . . not to mention phone calls you need to make or reports that must be submitted. To make matters worse, nowadays we get information from so many different sources—by phone, fax, and beeper, as well as all the mails—regular, voice, and electronic. It's no wonder we find it hard to keep track of it all. It's gotten to the point where psychologists have even coined a name for our experience in handling this glut of data: "information fatigue syndrome."

Fortunately, there are some wonderful devices out there that can help us remember. How do these memory tools work? By fulfilling the A.M. Principle. Memory tools get us to pay closer *attention* to information we need to remember, and they give that information *meaning* by placing it in an organizational scheme. In addition, they let us control what we need to remember by giving us the opportunity to review it.

You may already use a memory tool, such as an appointment book or a to-do list. However, there may be some memory maximizers that you don't use, or perhaps there are ways to use them more effectively. In this lesson, I'll explain why memory tools are so essential and how to get the most out of them.

## Why We Need Memory Tools

To me it seems as if there are so many reasons why memory tools are useful, it should go without saying that they are. However, I know that some of you may be skeptical, so here are my top five reasons:

**1. *Memory tools get us to pay attention to things we need to remember.*** Using a memory tool, just like using any technique to boost your brainpower, will focus your attention more actively on information you need to remember. Why? When we work with information, we pay closer attention to it.

Let's say you're at a planning meeting for your office holiday party. You have just agreed to order the decorations. Of course, everyone has an opinion about the party decor, but your boss rules the day with her suggestion of green and red palm trees and silver reindeer candles. You, though, are so busy thinking how nice purple balloons would look that you aren't really focused on what she is saying. When the group agrees to her idea you have no idea what they're talking about. Tough luck. If you had been using a memory tool such as Memory Minutes (discussed later in this step), you would have been paying closer attention to the discussion because you would have been taking notes, which you could review later at your own pace. Just by taking notes, you would have been paying closer attention.

**2. *Memory tools help us remember the things we need to remember but not memorize.*** We deal with three kinds of information:

- *Things we really need to remember.* This category includes certain things we *really* must remember, such as our name, address, phone number, PIN numbers, e-mail address, cell phone number, and the names of people we work with closely. Committing this kind of information to memory is essential.

- *Things we don't really need to remember.* Let's face it, there are some things we really, truly don't need to memorize. For example, if I need to call a restaurant for a reservation, I need to use that restaurant's phone number when I call, but I don't need to learn that phone number by heart (especially if I don't get a reservation).

- *Things we need to remember but not to memorize.* This is information we need to remember for a brief period of time to help us function effectively. Such information includes appointments, errands, and phone calls we have to make. In general, however, we do not need to commit this kind of information to long-term memory. For example, let's say you were taking a memory fitness class with me, and that class met every Wednesday night at 7:00 P.M. for eight weeks from February 4 to March 25. During the eight weeks of the class, you certainly would need to remember when and where the class was meeting (after all, it's pretty embarrassing to forget about your memory class). However, a year later, would you need to remember the class schedule? No.

If you think about it, most of the things we need to get along from day to day fall into the last category, things we need to remember for only a short time. Effort spent committing such information to long-term memory would be wasted, since this kind of information changes daily. You may wish to try it for mental exercise, but frankly, I can think of more exciting ways to give my brain a workout. Besides, isn't it worse to forget something you really need to do?

**3. *Memory tools help us control information.*** As we discussed in Step 2, many of us suffer from information overload. Not only is there more that we need to recall, but we have more sources of

---

### *Tools for Tables, Tools for Memory*

Still having trouble understanding why we need memory tools? Consider this analogy.

Let's say I asked you to build a table. What would you need? Probably material for the table, such as wood, in addition to tools, such as a hammer, a saw, and nails. Could you build that table without the tools, with your bare hands? Of course not— it would be too difficult to do that. Well, remembering everything you need to remember is a pretty tough task, as tough as building a piece of furniture. Tools that help us build our memory are just as essential as tools we use to build tables.

information to worry about. While before you may have received a letter, memo, or phone call about something you needed to do, today you get information in many more ways, including voice mail and e-mail. Most importantly, technology has increased the pace at which we receive information. Sometimes it's hard to keep up with it all. You already know that the best way to deal with information overload is to take control of the information. Organizational tools help us to do exactly that.

**4. *Memory tools get us organized.*** When we are organized, it's easier to find and remember the things that we need. We all know that life is easier when we have a system for placing and finding information. I often use the following example: Would it be easier to find a file labeled "Bobbins" in a cabinet where the files were arranged in alphabetical order or in one where they were just thrown in as they were made? The answer is rather obvious: Having the files in alphabetical order would make it easier to find the Bobbins file. It would also save you a lot of time and aggravation. One of my favorite stories of how helpful it is to organize information using memory tools comes from my client Sam S.:

> *Sam, a very successful businessman, was in his eighties and semiretired when we first met. When I asked Sam how he kept track of his appointments, he reached into his pocket and pulled out his wallet. Inside was a large pile of tattered yellow Post-it notes, each listing one appointment. As Sam showed me his system, several notes fell to the floor. No wonder he had trouble remembering his appointments! After a few sessions, Sam came in with a beautiful appointment book he'd received from his girlfriend. He got in the habit of using it and missed far fewer meetings.*

Memory tools allow us to organize information so it's easier for us to remember. Organizing information allows us to give it meaning, which, as we know, makes it more memorable.

**5. *Memory tools help us feel better.*** When we are organized we forget less and do more and generally are more effective and productive. Feeling effective is important to our self-esteem, since we feel better about ourselves when we see ourselves as capable. Being more productive means we are making the most of our time, so we have more time to do things we really want to do. This is how memory tools can help us feel better.

If these reasons are not convincing enough to you, let me add one more thought: If we don't need memory tools, then why do so many people use them?

## The Best Tools for Remembering What You Need to Do

Now that you know how important memory tools are, which ones should you be using? Here are the best tools you can use to organize information so that you can get things done.

### SCHEDULERS

Scheduling aids, such as appointment books, calendars, and electronic scheduling devices, are the most essential memory tools around. They help us keep track of things we need to remember—without them, let's face it, we'd be lost. How can you maximize your use of a scheduler? Here are a few tried-and-true tips:

• *Use a scheduling aid that fits your lifestyle.* Have you ever thought about how you keep track of your schedule? Do you buy the same appointment book year after year, without considering if it still

### Make a Memory Date

There are an enormous number of memory tools on the market today, from old-fashioned calendars and Rolodexes to computer organizer programs and digital voice-memo recorders. How can you figure out which memory tools will work best for you? Here's what I tell my clients: Make a memory date with yourself. Take a few hours to browse your local stationery store, office superstore, or office supply catalog. You'll find lots of new tools worth exploring and will be able to give yourself a chance to try them out. I always have fun on my memory dates and have found some really useful tools. So look in your appointment book and make a date to shop for some memory tools.

works for you or looking to see if something better is now on the market? Perhaps you just take the book or calendar the bank sends you and use that. Yes, it may seem to work, but are you really sure it's what you need? Consider this: If someone sent you a pair of glasses in the mail, would you use them? Of course not. After all, they probably wouldn't be the correct prescription and might not be your style. Well, your scheduling aid is as essential a tool for your memory as glasses are for your vision. You should devote as much attention and thought to choosing a scheduler as you would to choosing new spectacles.

One of the biggest obstacles to using a scheduler that suits you is falling into the habit of always using the same one. Many people use the same kind of book or calendar for years, regardless of changes in their lifestyle. I was guilty of this myself. Years ago, while on maternity leave, I never changed my appointment book to something that better suited my needs as a mother at home with small children; I continued to use the book I had needed when working. This, of course, meant that I never used my book, since it was totally impractical to carry it around in a diaper bag! As a result, I often "double booked" play dates and forgot doctors' appointments—all because I never thought about changing my scheduling aid. I've seen this happen with retirees as well. Retirement is a major life change, with concomitant changes in scheduling. Recent retirees understandably panic when they forget an appointment, but in most cases, their only memory problem is that they haven't yet adopted a good organizational technique suited to their new life.

How can you know if your scheduling aid fits your lifestyle? One clue is this: If you're not using it, it's probably not working for you! We tend not to use things that don't really suit us. The scheduler that you use should meet whatever your individual needs are for managing the information you need to remember daily. Your scheduling aid suits your lifestyle when it meets the following criteria:

- *It has enough room for you to write down all your appointments clearly.* You should be able to note the time of the appointment, the location (especially if it's not familiar to you), and the phone number of the person you are meeting or of the place you are going. That way you won't have to scramble for any information you may need at the last minute. This will also determine the size of your scheduler. If you have a very busy, active schedule you may need either a large appointment book or an electronic organizer, which can handle a lot of information. However, if you tend to make few appointments, you may be able to get away with using a smaller book (as long as it's one in which you can read the dates).

### The Electronic Age

If you despair that all technology has brought us is "information overload" and the stress that comes with it, take heart: The electronic age has also brought us some wonderful new tools to help manage that information. These include computerized scheduling programs, electronic organizers, voice-memo recorders, and more. All of these great inventions are available to help you be the master of your information domain. My favorite are the electronic organizers or personal data assistants (PDAs): They are small, lightweight, and can handle an enormous amount of information. You can keep in them not only your appointments but also addresses and notes. Several of the newer models synchronize with your desktop computer so that you can have a calendar there as well. Check them out on your memory date, and take advantage of all technology has to offer.

- *You can carry it with you most of the time.* Otherwise, you may not have it when you need it. I find that this is the single biggest reason why some people have two scheduling aids, such as a desk calendar at home and a small appointment book they carry with them. However, having two schedulers can be problematic, since you need to consolidate the information in them regularly or run the risk of confusing your schedule. While managing this way is not impossible (see "Double Planning" box, page 109), I still recommend using just one scheduling aid that you can carry with you most of the time. And don't let size discourage you: After all, many of us carry a briefcase or large bag that could easily accommodate a reasonably sized scheduler. If you're worried that you simply can't carry around a scheduler large enough for all your information, then try an electronic organizer.

• *Fill it in.* A scheduler can't help you if you don't put the information in it! Think of entering information into your scheduling aid as the acquisition step of memory: If you don't "get" it in, it's not going to be there later when you need it. Whether you make an appointment, get tickets to a concert series, or plan to meet someone at the movies, put it in your scheduler. Never, *never* depend on appointment cards, invitations, or newspaper clippings, which I guarantee you will either lose or not look at. Instead, keep a file folder or large envelope on your desk into which you place all loose notes, such as appointment cards and concert schedules. Then, as we'll see shortly, you can take the information from that folder or envelope and enter it into your scheduler during your Weekly Weigh-In.

• *Look for a scheduler that has a place for you to take short notes and keep frequently needed phone numbers.* While not absolutely necessary, it's very convenient to have room to jot notes in your scheduling aid as well as to have a place for phone numbers or fax numbers you often need.

In sum, a scheduling aid is one of the most important memory tools you can use. Get one that fits your lifestyle and use it.

## MASTER PLAN

How can you remember absolutely everything you have ever thought that you should do? Novels you always meant to read, vacations you want to plan, photos you want to reprint, project goals for career development? Write them down. Where? On what I call a Master Plan, a sheet of paper where you note absolutely everything you want to get done. It can be organized in any fashion you want—categorized by task, alphabetized, or listed by the WITOI-IWID ("When I Thought of It I Wrote It Down") Principle. Your Master Plan entries can range from the very simple, like "Send Rosie a birthday card," to the more complex, such as "Initiate new investment group." There is no time limit involved, since the goals on your Master Plan may be short- or long-range. The Master Plan is an effective memory tool because it acts as a reminder for all of those things that you plan to do but that may slip your mind. And it holds them all in one place, so you don't run the risk of losing the napkin on which you wrote that great screenplay idea, or of wallpapering your office with yellow sticky notes.

## TO-DO LIST
Another very important memory tool is your ordinary to-do list, which lists things you need to do. What are some of the best ways to use your to-do list?

• *Include everything you need to do over a certain period of time.* This includes errands, phone calls, or purchases that you can reasonably get done in a day or perhaps a week. I don't advise your including to-do-list chores that you can't achieve within that time frame. Why? Because you won't get it done, and all that will happen is that you'll feel lousy about not doing it. Items on your to-do list are drawn from your Master Plan and from your scheduler. Break down tasks that are too large into smaller, achievable steps. For example, don't put on your to-do list "Find cure for common cold." Chances are you won't get that done in a day or even a week. However, you could put down "Rent laboratory space" or "Buy tissues," since those are tasks you clearly could do in a week. Your lofty goal of curing colds really belongs on your Master Plan.

*Older and Wiser: The Telephone Appointment Study*
Researchers Morris Moscovitch and Nina Minde wanted to
see if there were age differences in how well people remembered things they had to do during the course of the day. To
test this, they asked two groups of subjects, one older and one
younger, to call an answering service at a specific time every
day for two weeks. (The older folks were similar in their level
of daily activity to their younger counterparts.) Of the nine people who missed their telephone appointments, only one was in
the older group. In fact, the researchers reported that the eight
younger subjects who forgot to phone in did so several times.
How did everyone in the older group remember so well? They
wrote down when they were supposed to call. In two further
variations on the telephone appointment study the investiga-
tors consistently found their older subjects remembered to call
in as well as or better than their younger peers. They concluded
that older adults were more concerned about forgetting, and
were therefore more likely to use a way to help themselves
remember. What does this prove? First, that memory tools
work. Second, that sometimes, older *is* wiser.

• *Organize it*. It's easier to use a to-do list that's organized. Like a
Master Plan, a to-do list can be organized in many ways, and many
preprinted to-do lists are available for purchase. I personally use a
loose sheet of paper and break my tasks into two categories: things
to do and phone calls, since most of my tasks can be divided in
that way. There's a sample to-do list on page 107—if you like it,
feel free to copy it and use it:

■ **THINGS TO DO** ■

*Day*: _____          *Date*: _____

CALLS:
*Who/Why:*                                  *Phone number:*

_____          _____

_____          _____

_____          _____

_____          _____

_____          _____

ERRANDS:

1. _____          7. _____
2. _____          8. _____
3. _____          9. _____
4. _____          10. _____
5. _____          11. _____
6. _____          12. _____

NOTES:

_____

_____

_____

_____

_____

_____

_____

_____

_____

• *Keep your to-do list in a place where you will see it.* A to-do list just works better when you can find it! I keep my to-do list in my scheduler at the page for the current date.

• *When you finish a task on your to-do list, cross it off!* Why? Because it feels good—and it will remind you that you've done it!

## The Best Habits for Remembering What You Need to Do

So you've gotten the perfect scheduling aid, written out your Master Plan, and started a to-do list. Now what? Clearly, just *having* tools to help us organize what we need to remember isn't enough. In addition to finding these tools, we need to use them, and use them in a way that maximizes their power. Here are some helpful habits:

### THE WEEKLY WEIGH-IN

At the beginning of every week, either Sunday evening or Monday morning, take five minutes to "weigh in." Sit down with your scheduling aid, Master Plan, and to-do list. First, go through your schedule for the upcoming week. Take the file folder or envelope in which you've put papers with information you need, and enter that information into your scheduler now. Make sure you put everything in your scheduler, including the addresses of any unfamiliar places you must go, phone numbers, and anything else you may need. Once the information is entered, throw away the piece of paper it came on (unless of course you really need it, in which case you can put it in your tickler file, described on page 116). Figure out what you need to do for any of the items on your schedule for that week, and put those things on your to-do list. Also transfer unfinished items from

---

### Double Planning

I know many people are devoted to using two schedulers, a large one at home or at work and then another smaller one they carry with them. While I usually advise against this arrangement, here's a tip for making it work: Make sure you cross-reference your two schedulers during your Daily Grind and Weekly Weigh-In. That way you'll ensure that the same information is in both schedulers. Or you could forgo a smaller book and instead write your daily schedule on a separate piece of paper with your to-do list. That way you can have one book but keep your schedule for that day with you. If you make any appointments during the day, you can make a note of it on your daily list and transfer the information to your scheduler later. Many preprinted lists include a place for your schedule and things you need to do, plus have room for notes. If you're a double planner, look for them on your memory date.

---

your last to-do list to this new one. Next, look at your Master Plan and add to your to-do list any tasks from that list that you need to do or will have time to do in the upcoming week. Once finished, you've weighed in and are ready to start a very organized week.

## THE DAILY GRIND

Every morning—or the evening before, if that suits you better—take a moment to look at your scheduler and to-do list. If you make it a habit to look at these tools every day at least once, you will be focusing your attention on what you need to do and will be giving yourself an opportunity to review it. So, have a little Daily Grind with your morning coffee or tea—it will do wonders for your memory!

If you use the tools—a scheduling aid, Master Plan, and to-do list—and practice the habits—the Weekly Weigh-In and Daily Grind—I promise you will be amazed at how well you remember the things you need to do.

## How to Remember What Was Said

Ever have trouble recalling details from an important conversation? Information you receive at a doctor's appointment is a great example of this. You meet with your doctor briefly. During that time, she examines you and tells you what she thinks is going on and what she wants you to do about it. Perhaps you need to schedule some tests or take certain medications. All that information in so little time! And what happens? You wake up at 3:00 A.M. with a funny feeling in your stomach and you can't remember if that was one of the side effects she told you to look out for. You're really worried, but too embarrassed to call the doctor in the middle of the night. Well, let's face it, how could you possibly recall everything she said? After all, you heard it so quickly, and were probably distracted to boot when she was talking to you, given that you weren't feeling well and were anxious about the diagnosis.

### MEMORY MINUTES

What can you do to help yourself remember what was said? The best way to remember a conversation is to take notes, or what I call Memory Minutes. Remember taking classes in high school or college? How would you keep track of the information in a lecture or seminar presentation? Chances are you took notes. Yet how often do you do that now? Probably not very often, if you're like most people I meet. That's too bad, because using Memory Minutes is a great way to help yourself recall that information more effectively. Why?

• *Memory Minutes get you to focus more actively on what is being said.* There are many times when we're hearing something we really need to remember but we are distracted. In this situation, take Memory Minutes. Write down for yourself the information you need to remember. Then, when you wake up at 3:00 A.M., you can just look at your notes and see whether or not that stomach pain is something your doctor said to worry about.

• *Memory Minutes give you control over information.* When you write something down you've mastered it. You can review it at your own pace, going back to it as often as you need to. One of my favorite stories about Memory Minutes illustrates this:

> *Jane W., a fifty-two-year-old psychologist, came to class very frustrated and upset that she couldn't remember anything. She said she was taking over the treasurer position of her block association and was having trouble getting a handle on the information that the previous treasurer was passing on to her. There seemed to be gaps in the information, and when she spoke with him about it he said she was forgetting things he'd already told her. After some discussion, the class agreed that Jane should try taking Memory Minutes during her conversations with the previous treasurer. The next week, Jane walked in smiling. She'd taken notes as we had discussed, and realized that her memory was just fine. It was the information she was getting that had holes in it!*

---

*"The strongest memory is not as good as the weakest ink."*
— CONFUCIUS

Feel free to take Memory Minutes any way you wish. Some of my clients keep a separate spiral-bound notebook for each doctor. You may prefer to take notes on loose paper and later file them in an appropriate folder. It doesn't matter how you do it, just do it. Memory Minutes will definitely improve your effectiveness in remembering what was said.

## How to Remember Where Things Are

Sometimes we need help remembering where we put things. Most of us have at one time or another lost our keys, glasses, checkbook, or that piece of paper we had just a second ago. Have you ever stopped to think about why we misplace these items so often? Usually it's because we aren't paying attention when we put them down. We're distracted, and putting something down is not what we're focusing on. Misplacing things has nothing to do with how old we are—only with how busy. Take the following story about my friend Carla:

*Carla, a busy massage therapist in her early thirties, once called me, quite distraught because she had lost her wallet. The last time she remembered having it was when she was paying a taxi driver. At the time, she was carrying a bunch of packages, so she figured she must have dropped her wallet either in the cab or on the street. After commiserating, we agreed that she should cancel her credit cards and call her customers who'd given her checks that day so that they could stop payment on them. About two weeks later, Carla called again. She'd found her wallet. Where? Seems that when she walked in the door with all those packages, she put her wallet down in the first convenient place, which happened to be on the top of a bookcase. Since she was preoccupied with all her packages, Carla wasn't paying atten-*

*tion when she put her wallet in that unusual spot. She found it only because she was cleaning. While Carla was happy to have her wallet back, she was pretty frustrated by all she'd been through for simply not paying attention.*

## FORGET-ME-NOT SPOT

How can we prevent ourselves losing things we need and save ourselves the aggravation, not to mention wasted time, that goes along with it? The best way to remember where things are is to always put them in the same place, what I like to call a forget-me-not spot. Why? In Step 1, I introduced the "overlearning paradox"—the fact that the more we do something, the less attention we have to pay to it. Well, we can apply overlearning to help rev up our recall for where we put things. If we always put the items we need, such as our wallet, keys, and glasses, in the same place, we don't need to pay attention to where we put them, as they will always be in that forget-me-not spot. Here are some tips for using a forget-me-not spot:

• *Pick a convenient place.* Your forget-me-not spot should be conveniently located so you will really use it. At home, I think the best place is near the door you use most frequently. At your office, the best place is most likely somewhere on your desk.

• *Make sure it can hold all your things.* Your forget-me-not spot should be something that can hold the objects you want to put

> *"I got it all together but forgot where I put it."*
> —FROM A PILLOW I SAW IN SOMEONE'S HOME

there. It can be a drawer, a shelf, a bowl on a tabletop, or a box. I once heard about a woman who had a table in her foyer painted with images of her keys, wallet, and glasses. While it probably worked well, it's not really necessary to go to so much trouble! Plain or fancy, make sure your forget-me-not spot can fit all the objects you need it to. It's also nice if there's extra room for small items you may need to remember to take someplace, such as a book you need to return to the library or dry-cleaning receipts.

• *Get into the habit of using your forget-me-not spot.* If a forget-me-not spot is going to work for you, you really need to use it. This really is a case of use it or lose it!

---

### ■ HOT TIP ■
#### *Nag Notes*

Keep a package of sticky notes in your forget-me-not spot. That way, when you remember an errand you need to run or something you need to do, you can make a note and stick it on the door. You'll see it on your way out and it will serve as a timely reminder. Some experts recommend putting whatever you need to take with you in front of the door. I have two concerns with this: First, unless you live alone, chances are someone else will move whatever it is out of their way if they leave home first. Second, I always worry that someone will trip over their dry cleaning or umbrella on the way out. So try writing yourself a nag note and putting it on the door instead.

---

---

*Memory Tools to Remember*

| | |
|---|---|
| Schedulers | Electronic organizers |
| Personal data assistants | White boards |
| Master Plan | Digital memo recorders |
| To-do lists | Memory Minutes |
| Perpetual calendars | Tickler files |
| Address books | Checklists |
| Forget-me-not spot | Nag notes |
| Locator logs | Medication boxes |

---

## More Great Memory Tools

Here are some other tools that help organize information so it's more memorable:

### ADDRESS BOOKS

Many of us have a book or Rolodex in which we keep addresses and phone numbers that are important to us. However, when was the last time you updated yours? My husband still treasures his address book from sixth grade. Unfortunately, it doesn't have room left for new addresses, not to mention space for fax numbers and e-mail addresses. Think about how well your current address book is working for you. Perhaps it's time for a change. You may want to consider keeping your address book in electronic form, especially if you have a lot of address information to keep or need to update it regularly. There are several good software programs you can use to manage addresses. If you like to carry your address book with you, consider an electronic organizer. Most come with address managers in addition to scheduling programs, giving you double the work for half the weight.

## PERPETUAL CALENDARS

Here's another great tool I discovered on a recent memory date. A perpetual calendar is a calendar that is not referenced to any particular year, so you can use it to keep track of birthdays and anniversaries. At the beginning of the year, when you get a new scheduling aid, you can take your perpetual calendar and enter those important dates into your schedule for that year. If you really want to show off, look at your perpetual calendar at the beginning of every month and get those birthday and anniversary cards out on time.

## TICKLER FILES

Often we have information or papers we don't need right away but will need eventually. Concert tickets, school schedules for next year, and invitations fall into this category. Rather than stuffing all of these things into a drawer and then ransacking the drawer for them a few minutes before you need them, try putting them into a tickler file. A tickler file is a filing system devoted to maintaining information you will need in the future. One of the best tickler filing systems is to have a file designated for each month of the year. You can then file items according to the month you need them. Season tickets to the local team's baseball games? When you get them, note the dates and times in your scheduler, and then file the tickets by month in your tickler files. Believe me, spending a few minutes using a tickler file really beats spending even more time getting frustrated when you can't find things later. You'll be tickled pink at the time and aggravation you save.

## CHECKLISTS AND WHITE BOARDS

Remember the energy crisis in the 1970s? All around America, light switches were adorned with cute reminders to turn off the lights and conserve energy (in fact, you can still find some of those stickers around the medical center where I work). Those stickers prompted us to remember to do something. You can help yourself remember something you have to do by writing yourself a note and leaving it in an appropriate place. A checklist is very helpful for remembering a sequence of related tasks that may be difficult to remember and/or infrequently performed. For example, if you have trouble remembering how to record a TV show on your VCR, make a checklist of the steps you need to follow and leave it next to your TV. Chances are that having a checklist will help you learn the task better as you practice it.

White boards (erasable boards made of a smooth white plastic material) come in all sizes and are available at most office supply or stationery stores. They're great to have on the back of a door or on the refrigerator to jot a note to yourself about something you must do. Write yourself great big notes and erase them often so that you don't stop paying attention to the board.

---

■ HOT TIP ■
### *Family Planning*

Here's a great tip for busy families: Get a white-board calendar and put it in the kitchen or family room. Assign each family member a different-color pen and write their activities, such as soccer games and school plays, in the squares for the appropriate days. We do it in our home and have found that it's one of the best ways to keep track of everyone's schedules. If your children are older, it's fun to do this as a family so that everyone gets to be a part of the action.

---

## LOCATOR LOGS

Ever have trouble remembering that very safe place where you hid your jewelry, birth certificate, PIN code, or insurance documents? It's frequently hard for us to recall exactly where these important papers or valuable items are because we like to put them in protected, out-of-the-way locations. Also, since such items are rarely used, we aren't constantly reminded of their location. The solution? Take this tip from my very organized student Yvette: Keep a locator log. Using an address book, record each important item and its "address." For example, when you put your extra house keys in the tea canister, turn to the "K" in your locator log and note that the keys are located there. That way you can locate them when necessary with no muss, fuss, or additional aggravation.

## MEDICATION BOXES

Medication boxes are the best way to store medication that you need to take. They come in all sizes and shapes, some as simple as a rectangular plastic box with three compartments for time of day, while others hold a month's supply of pills. By putting your medication in the box so it is organized by when you must take it, you will be more likely to remember to take your medications properly. Also—and for some of us even more important—a medication box can help you remember whether or not you've taken your medication. I strongly prefer them over pillboxes, where different medications can easily get confused, and it can be very difficult to recall whether a medication has been taken. While younger people often dismiss medication boxes, they are really worth considering. After all, too many of us forget to finish an antibiotic prescription or to take our vitamins.

## HUMAN RESOURCES

We frequently rely on others to remember certain information. For example, in our household (as much as I might hate to admit it)

> *"The darkest secret in the lives of Americans is that their memories are failing. It's not just an age problem— it is something every person, regardless of advancing years, has dealt with. We all live in fear that someone else will find out about us, when in fact that someone else can't remember anything, either."*
> —ART BUCHWALD

my husband remembers the trash collection schedule. I can take out the newspapers on Wednesdays as well as anyone else, but heaven help us if I'm the one who has to remember that's the day they go out. Of course, the same is true in reverse, since my husband often relies on me to remember family birthdays and weekend plans.

Many of us depend on others to hold information for us without even realizing it.

*Howard M. came to see me several years ago, terrified that he was losing his memory. Then seventy-nine years old, Howard had retired from his work as a successful business consultant two years earlier. Retirement for this gentleman meant that he worked forty hours a week instead of seventy and had dismissed his assistant, who'd been with him for twenty-three years. In our initial consultation, I asked Howard what kinds of things he'd been forgetting. "Well," he said, "just yesterday I forgot where I was supposed to meet a client for lunch. And last week I made it to a meeting, but left the papers I needed at my office." As we discussed these memory lapses further, I inquired how Howard had managed that kind of information in the* past. "Why, my assistant took care of it, of course," he replied. You see, Howard, while brilliant, was quite disorganized, and had been for most of his life. The problem he was having wasn't that he suddenly was forgetting details he'd always remembered in the past, but rather that he'd taken responsibility for keeping track of things he'd never had to keep track of before, since his assistant had always done it. As a result of our consultation, Howard rehired his assistant part-time. The last time we spoke, he was happily consulting and leaving the organizational details to her.

Remember that it's okay to have other people remember things for you. You shouldn't be embarrassed to ask someone to remind you about something you've forgotten. Certainly they forget things as well sometimes.

---

## ■ HOT TIP ■
### I Leave Myself a Message

Here's a tip from Joyce, a former student of mine. When Joyce, a working mom with a busy catering business, is really concerned that she may forget something she has to do, she leaves herself a message on her answering machine. Depending on the task, she'll leave it on either her home or office service. I've tried this myself a few times when I couldn't make a note of something and was concerned I'd forget it. It really works!

---

# Ten Top Tips for Getting Organized

We've covered the most important information to help you boost your brainpower with memory tools. Here are ten more great tips to help you get organized:

### 1  Use a filing system effectively.

Take the time to think through your filing system. Figure out what organization will work best for you—client files versus project files, color coding, and so on. Once you've worked out your system, make sure to use it. File all pertinent information in the appropriate file (not a desk pile). It's also helpful to attach blank sheets of paper to the inside right back flap of file folders. Then, you can take notes on relevant conversations, memos, and meetings right where you need them. And make sure you put your files away in an organized fashion!

### 2  Use a task list for projects.

Overwhelmed by a complex project? Think through the project concretely, step by step. Then, make a list for all these steps, or tasks, to help you get them done. Here's another suggestion: Keep your task list stapled to the inside front cover of your project file. That way you can refer to the task list whenever you work on that project.

### 3  Avoid paper piles.

Are you surrounded by a sea of papers at work? Is your dining-room table so covered with mail that you're not even sure it's still there? There are generally two things that happen to information buried in a paper pile—either it is forgotten or it can't be found when you need it. Paper piles are like the plague—they should be avoided at all costs. When you get a piece of paper, you should do one of three things: file it, write the information down elsewhere (such as in your scheduler) and toss it, or simply toss it.

4 **Avoid constantly putting information on sticky notes and other small pieces of paper.**
If you need to write something down, put it on your Master Plan or on your to-do list. While it's okay to use a reminder such as a sticky note every once in a while, using such notes all the time will make them less noticeable and—as a result—less useful.

5 **Organize your day according to your energy level.**
Most of us are at our best in the morning. Therefore, set aside time in the morning to work on projects that require your full focus and ability. Schedule less important meetings and other tasks for later in the day.

6 **Stick to your plan.**
The best-laid plans often fall victim to their makers. While spontaneity is important, there is a fine line between it and simple procrastination. Once you've come up with a good strategy for tackling a task, stay with it. Only you can prevent yourself from dillydallying.

7 **Help yourself avoid interruption.**
Ever had one of those days where nothing seemed to get done? Often we are unable to complete tasks because we get distracted. In order to get things done, you must protect your time. If possible, leave your phone on voice mail during times you have scheduled to work on projects. If you have a private office, close your

door. You could even put up a sign saying something like "Hard at Work: Please Come Back Later." If you are interrupted, help keep the disruption brief by remaining task-oriented.

**8** **Schedule time to make phone calls and return e-mail.**
When you leave a phone message, include times that you will be available by phone. Ask the other party to do the same—it will save you both a lot of time that would otherwise be spent on everyone's favorite game, phone tag. Also, avoid checking your voice mail and e-mail constantly. Instead, review them at scheduled intervals during the day.

**9** **Schedule stress breaks during the day.**
Make sure you give yourself a break! Working to the point of total brain fatigue and muscle tension will never do you any good. Stretch, take some deep breaths, go out to get your lunch, call your kids—do something to give yourself a little break. If you'd like, you can schedule these breaks as a reward for when you've completed a specific task.

**10** **Appreciate your own style.**
Just as we are all different in other ways, we all have different organizational styles. Remember that you have gotten where you are today because of who you are and what you have accomplished. Use improved organizational skills to enhance your personal style, not change it. Getting organized should make you feel good, not burdened.

You can get more information on organizational techniques from sources devoted to organizational management. Some of these experts focus on organizing your life to meet your values and goals, not only your appointments. Look in the self-help section of your local bookstore for further information on getting organized.

Using memory tools to help you organize information you need to remember is a great way to maximize your memory fitness. You will remember better if you are using the right tools for you and practicing the best memory habits for using them.

■ STEP 4: QUIZ ■

*This quiz will help organize the information in this lesson. Answer the following questions "true" or "false" (answers appear on page 126).*

**T F**   1 A forget-me-not spot is a place I can go to remember.

**T F**   2. A scheduling aid should suit one's lifestyle.

**T F**   3. The "Daily Grind" refers to the time each day when I look at my appointment book and to-do list to remind myself of what I need to do that day.

**T F**   4. Organizational aids are tools that can help me remember more effectively.

**T F**   5. I will be more likely to forget information if I write it down instead of trying to memorize it.

**T F**   6. We often look to other people as resources to help us remember information.

**T F**   7. To remember my appointments for the week, I should look at them on Monday and memorize them all at once.

**T F**   8. A locator log is a tool I can use to help me keep track of my children.

**T F**   9. Recorded minutes of important conversations and events allow me to have more control over the information I have gotten.

**T F**  10. A to-do list can help remind me of errands and tasks I need to get done.

■ STEP 4: ANSWERS ■

1. **False.** *A forget-me-not spot is a location where you always keep important objects that you frequently need (e.g., keys, wallet, glasses) when they are not in use.*

2. **True.** *A scheduling aid is an essential tool for organizing information you need to remember. It should suit your lifestyle so you will be able to use it most effectively. Let's face it, if it doesn't really work for you, you're not going to use it!*

3. **True.** *Practicing the habit of a Daily Grind will give you a chance to review your daily schedule and tasks so that you will be more likely to remember them.*

4. **True.** *Organizational aids are tools, not crutches. Anyone who has a lot of information to manage, no matter what their age, can benefit from their use.*

5. **False.** *Writing things down is an effective way to remember them. Having such information in writing allows you to review it again and gives you control over the information.*

6. **True.** *We frequently have others in our lives whom we can turn to for recalling certain kinds of information — such as the trash collection schedule and birthdays of family members.*

7. **False.** *While you should look at your appointments for the week during your Weekly Weigh-in on Monday (or Sunday evening), you should never attempt to memorize all your appointments, unless you feel doing so is fun! That's what your scheduling aid is for.*

8. **False.** *A locator log is a device you can use to keep track of where you keep important items, such as extra keys, important documents,*

*or jewelry. You'll have to think of another way to keep track of your children!*

**9. True.** *Memory Minutes allow you to go back over the information at your own pace and as frequently as you need to in order to learn it.*

**10. True.** *A to-do list is an excellent tool for keeping track of things you must get done.*

■ **STEP 4: MEMORCISES** ■

**1.** Get yourself organized! Choose a scheduling aid that best meets your needs. Enter into it all your appointments and other necessary information.

**2.** Over the next week, get in the habit of doing the Daily Grind and Weekly Weigh-In.

**3.** Start using a to-do list.

**4.** Figure out where your forget-me-not spot will be and what will go in it. Then, *use it consistently,* especially for those items you often misplace.

**5.** Start keeping Memory Minutes for important conversations and events. Title each entry for easy access, using the date, topic, and names of people involved.

# STEP

## 5

# Train Your Brain

■ IN THIS STEP YOU WILL LEARN: ■

*What Internal Memory Techniques Are*
*How Internal Memory Techniques Work*
*Eight Memory Techniques You Can Really Use*

By now you understand that there are many ways to maximize our memory fitness. We can improve our attention to things we want to remember so we learn more of what we need to recall. We can be aware of issues in our lifestyle that interfere with our memory performance and deal with them more effectively to lessen their impact. We can use tools to help us organize information we need to retain so we can function at our best.

What if, however, you find yourself in a situation where you really need or want to remember something despite the disruptions of life and without the use of tools? Perhaps you want to recall a list of talking points for a major presentation and would prefer not to use notes. Or you see a "for sale" sign on a car you'd like to check out but don't have a pen to write down the phone number. Situations like those require another way to get the information so that

---

### *Why I Don't Use the Term "Mnemonics"*

The techniques taught in this lesson are frequently referred to as "mnemonics." The term *mnemonic* (taken from the name of the Greek goddess of memory, Mnemosyne) actually refers to *anything* you use to help yourself remember, including calendars, files, and relaxing if necessary. Everything taught in this book would therefore qualify as a mnemonic. However, I avoid using the term since many people regard mnemonics as less-than-reputable "tricks" to improve memory. Instead I prefer to call my methods "internal memory techniques."

---

you can remember it later. This lesson will introduce techniques to help you remember information "by head" (after all, it's not your heart that does the work!).

## What Internal Memory Techniques Are

Using a technique to help us learn something we want to remember is another way we can make the most of our memory. Internal memory techniques have been around for centuries, so long in fact that one researcher was prompted to call memory improvement "one of the world's oldest professions." The ancient Greeks wrote extensively about the use of internal memory techniques, many of which are the same methods employed today. Performers who demonstrate feats of memory use such techniques to wow audiences with their skill.

Why, then, have so many people found these techniques frustrating and, quite frankly, more of a hindrance than a help? Actually, the problem is not with the techniques themselves, but rather with the way in which they have been taught. Memory improvement experts in the past have offered memory systems that are difficult to learn and burdensome to use. Methods such as the peg or loci technique are great for people who want "super" memories. However, they really aren't that helpful for the average person. Most of us don't have hours to spend learning a complex internal memory system before we can use it. And let's be honest: Are you really that concerned with remembering *absolutely* everything? Probably not, if you're like me and most people I know. You'd just like to remember *better*.

If you've struggled with memory improvement in the past, you will be relieved that the approach to internal memory techniques taught here is quite different. After all, this program is not about a special ploy for memory improvement. I don't believe that there is only one, best way to make more of your memory. So you will not be learning a single memory system here. Rather, this lesson will introduce you to several simple, practical techniques you can use to rev up your recall for information. I offer different techniques so you can find a method that best suits your personality and lifestyle. Why? If a technique is not simple, you'll never learn it. If it's not practical, you'll never turn to it when you need it. And if it doesn't feel right for you, you will never get into the habit of using it.

Do we need internal memory techniques to improve our memory? Not necessarily. You can improve your memory by being attentive to information you need to remember, by identifying and coping effectively with things in your daily life that limit your memory potential, and by practicing good organizational habits. However, I often advise my clients to make at least one internal memory technique part of their memory fitness routine, since there are circumstances where they are useful. For example, you may need to remember something "by head," such as a license plate number, a cell phone number, or a PIN number. Or you may find yourself in

## The Science of It All . . .

While memory improvement techniques such as the ones taught in this step have been around for centuries, many people question whether they actually work. Some of those people, of course, are researchers, who have looked extensively at the effectiveness of internal memory techniques. In general, research on internal memory techniques has found that such methods do work. However, scientists have found that memory improvement is limited to the area on which you are working, and doesn't generalize to all aspects of your memory function. In other words, using a specific technique to improve memory in one area won't necessarily help recall in another. Also, research suggests that simply learning an internal memory technique once doesn't mean it will help you down the road. What does this all mean? First, that internal memory techniques are not the only thing necessary for improved memory fitness. Second, that memory techniques will only work for you if you use them.

a situation where you don't have much control over the information and need to absorb it quickly. This is often the case when you're getting directions or learning a name.

Finally, part of what makes this program unique is the realization that, when it comes to improving your memory, schemes for memorizing information are not enough. Having a better memory is the result of improving your overall memory fitness. You can hang information on "pegs" in your head from now until the year 2050, but if you don't take good care of yourself and can't organize worth beans, you still will forget. A good internal memory technique can be an important part of better memory fitness. However, it is not a substitute for it.

## How Internal Memory Techniques Work

Internal memory techniques are very powerful ways to learn and remember information. In large part this is due to the fact that they fulfill the A.M. Principle. Let's look at how they work:

• *They force you to focus* **attention** *on what you are trying to learn.* When you apply an internal memory technique, you are forced to concentrate. In fact, just using a technique makes it impossible *not* to pay attention. And we already know that we absorb something we want to remember more effectively when we attend to it.

• *They give* **meaning** *to what you are trying to learn.* Internal memory techniques are successful because they give meaning to something you want to remember. This works in two ways: In many cases, we can find meaning inherent to the information we are trying to learn. Or we can impose meaning on material that doesn't necessarily have that meaning to make it more memorable. And something that is meaningful is more memorable.

Some of you may believe internal memory techniques are simply too complicated for you. If so, think again. Chances are you already use some of these methods without even knowing it. Take a look at these examples:

- What year did Columbus sail for America? Did you say 1492? That's correct. Chances are you got there by reciting the following rhyme: *"In 1492, Columbus sailed the ocean blue."* Rhymes such as these are a popular internal memory technique.

- How can you remember the correct spelling of the word "stationery"? Well, if in fourth grade you learned the saying, *"Stationery is for a letter,"* you were given a way of connecting the correct spelling of stationery with another word you already knew the proper spelling for. English teachers loved these connection techniques for learning proper spelling.

- Here's one from the history books. Need to remember what happened to the wives of Henry VIII? Perhaps someone taught you the following rhyme for recalling their fates: *Divorced, beheaded, died; divorced, beheaded, survived.*

- Trying to remember the colors of the rainbow? Consider the following first letter association, which my son learned in his kindergarten class: *ROY G. BIV.* This name is made up of the first letter of each color in the rainbow: red, orange, yellow, green, blue, indigo, and violet.

You can see from these examples that internal memory techniques are really part of our everyday world. So don't be afraid of these methods. They can be simple to learn and use, and can help you remember better.

The goal of this step is to help you learn an internal memory technique that you like and will use. There is no reason for you to be a memory dilettante, practicing a myriad of internal memory methods. Just figure out which one of these techniques suits you, and do it. This step will work best for you if you:

1. *Read through all the techniques.* Some of them are similar, some of them are very different. Some will seem as easy as pie; others will appear impossible and you'll be tempted to skip them.

Don't. Think about each one and consider whether it feels like something you could do.

2. *Use the first set of exercises to try all the techniques.* In the Memorcises for this step, you'll find two sets of exercises. Use the first set to practice all the different methods described. Perhaps using the Snapshot Technique is easier than you first thought. Or maybe you'll uncover a hidden talent for the First Letter Association Technique. Make sure you use *all* the methods on *all* the exercises in that first set—that way, you'll be able to compare how well they work for you.

3. *Use the second set of exercises to practice your favorite technique.* Now you're ready to pick your favorite internal memory technique. Practice your method using the second set of exercises.

4. *Make your internal memory technique part of your overall memory fitness program.* You're ready to add your favorite internal memory method to your daily routine. Use it daily, practicing on information you don't really need to remember as well as on stuff you want to learn "by head." Making your favorite internal memory technique a habit means that it will be working for you when you really need it. As we all know, practice makes perfect (or at least close to it!).

One final note: This step introduces you to several internal memory techniques that are simple to learn and practical to use. These methods can be applied to many different types of information that need to be remembered. In this way they are distinct from the techniques you will find in Steps 6 and 7, which focus on methods for remembering specific kinds of information. Of course, since the methods presented here work well with all kinds of information, you will note some overlap between what you learn in this step and in those that follow. You may find that you prefer the same or similar techniques in both steps. This will give you a great advantage in getting a good internal memory habit under your belt.

# Eight Memory Techniques You Can Really Use

Ready to learn about some great internal memory techniques? Here are eight methods guaranteed to boost your brainpower:

### 1 The Repetition Technique

Here's a technique so simple you probably do it already and don't even think about the fact that you're using a method to help yourself remember. When you need to learn something "by head," repeat it to yourself. By repeating the information, you are getting yourself to focus attention on it and thus giving yourself more opportunity to learn it. Sometimes that's all it takes.

### 2 The Link Technique

One powerful way we can remember better is by hooking together the information we are trying to learn. I often refer to this in class as a "dominoes" technique. Like a series of dominoes knocking one another down in a line, you can remember items by linking them one to another. Take the following list of randomly selected words:

**table**

**pen**

**locket**

**umbrella**

**salt**

To link this list, I first hook "table" to "pen." Perhaps I see a pen on a table, or think about a table shaped like a pen. Next, I connect "pen" with "locket." Maybe I visualize a pen with a locket on a chain wrapped around it or a pen hanging from someone's neck like a locket. Following that, I hook "locket" to "umbrella." I could picture another locket shaped like an umbrella, or perhaps an outdoor market cart selling trinkets, with the word "lockets" written in large letters on the umbrella. Finally, I link "umbrella" to "salt," perhaps by picturing the Morton Salt container, with the image of the little girl protecting herself from the rain of salt with an umbrella. Now I have linked this list: When I think of "table," it will remind me of "pen." "Pen" will trigger my recollection of "locket," "locket" will lead me to "umbrella," and "umbrella" will help me recall "salt." I have successfully used this simple technique to learn and remember this word list.

The Link Technique is a great way to learn and remember information, especially if that information lends itself to being hooked together. It is one of the simpler and more straightforward techniques, as it doesn't require a great deal of creative energy or time. It is particularly powerful when used for lists, as we shall see in Step 6.

### 3 The Storytelling Technique

If you want to remember something, make up a story about it. Storytelling is a wonderful way to make information memorable. It not only connects the information together, but also gives it narrative meaning. For most of us, a story is an easy thing to recall.

Let's say that you want to memorize the following license plate number:

**N M 1 2 0 F**

Making up a story involving the information in the license plate number can help you do that. My story for this license plate is: "In New Mexico, it's 120 degrees Fahrenheit." Now we'll be able to use that story to help us remember the license plate more effectively.

Storytelling is also a great general memory technique because it's very versatile. It's easy to make up a story about something as simple as a license plate number or as complicated as points in a presentation. Let's say you had to memorize the ingredients for a favorite chicken dish (it would probably be best to write it down, but let's just try this one for fun). You need:

> **chicken**
> **chicken broth**
> **wild rice**
> **dried apples**
> **walnuts**
> **salt**
> **pepper**

How can you remember this list? Make up a story. Here's mine:

> A chicken went walking through a wild-rice paddy. The paddy soon smelled like chicken broth. On the other side it ended up in an apple orchard full of old dried apples. Next it ended up in a walnut grove. It made the farmer so upset his hair turned salt and pepper.

Storytelling is one of the more involved techniques presented here, since it requires some imagination and time to use. However, I find that this is one of the most popular techniques I teach, since we are all familiar with stories and tend to like them. Storytelling is my favorite internal memory technique; perhaps it will be yours as well. We'll learn more about storytelling and lists such as this one in the next step.

## 4  The Connection Technique

Another simple way to make something more memorable is to give it meaning by connecting what you are learning to something that you already know. Many people find that they naturally make a connection between newly learned material and something known to them beforehand. Let's use a number I once had to memorize as an example. When the medical center where I work changed the phone system, I had to learn the following access code:

$$7 \; 6 \; 9 \; 0 \; 1 \; 3$$

In order to remember this number, I came up with the following connection: The first two digits, 76, reminded me of a song from one of my favorite musicals, *Music Man*. Humming "Seventy-six trombones led the big parade . . ." I made a connection to the next two numbers, 9 and 0. I park at a garage on 90th Street, so I coupled these numbers to that familiar location. Finally, I found I could remember the next two digits, 1 and 3, by hooking them to my son's birthday, which falls on the thirteenth of the month. By making a connection between this number and information already known to me, I was able to learn and remember it more effectively.

The Connection Technique allows you to take advantage of information you already have and use it to give meaning to something newly learned, thereby making that information more memorable. The Connection Technique is a wonderful way to learn names, as we shall see in Step 7. If you aren't really comfortable with more complex internal memory methods, try this one.

### 5 The Rhyme Technique

Many people like to help themselves remember information by making up a rhyme for it. While the Rhyme Technique requires a lot of creative energy and a certain talent, my students who like it *really* like it. They find it fun to make up rhymes—and, let's face it, if something's fun, you're more likely to do it. How does the Rhyme Technique work? Let's take the recipe list from above again, only this time let's try to learn it using this technique:

chicken

chicken broth

wild rice

dried apples

walnuts

salt

pepper

Here's a rhyme to help you remember this list of ingredients:

Oh, the chicken swam into the broth

The rice brewed wildly

The apples dried on walnut husks

On the salt and pepper sea.

If you are musically inclined, you may even find you like to give your rhymes a little tune. Some students who are musicians or composers enjoy the Rhyme Technique. While it may seem complicated, make sure to try it. Maybe you'll uncover an unknown talent!

### 6 First Letter Association Technique

The First Letter Association Technique is another familiar method, where you take the first letter of each word in a list of words you wish to remember and make a word or phrase associating to it. Abbreviations and acronyms are popular examples of first letter association. Take the following examples:

- *What does U.S.A. stand for?* If you said United States of America, you're correct (and you thought these techniques were hard!).

- *What does TGIF mean?* "Thank God It's Friday," a popular refrain.

- *Do you know the names of the five Great Lakes?* Chances are you do, but it may be a bit hard to think of them. If you remember the first letter association HOMES, however, you'll always be able to think of them: Huron, Ontario, Michigan, Erie, and Superior.

Why are first letter associations so popular? Most likely because they are such a powerful way for us to remember things. Let's look at why:

1. *First letter associations get us to focus attention and give meaning to material we are learning.* Like other internal memory techniques, first letter associations help us fulfill the A.M. Principle.

2. *First letter associations allow us to remember more by memorizing less.* When we use a first letter association we reduce the material we must memorize. Since the technique takes the first letter of each item on a list and makes a meaningful word or acronym from those letters, it significantly shortens the amount of information you need to commit to memory. Take the above example of using the word HOMES to help recall the names of the five Great Lakes. When you recall that one word it reminds you of the five names you need.

3. *First letter associations give us clues.* It's always easier to recall information when you have a little help doing so. First letter associations give us the first letter for whatever it is we are trying to remember. That first letter acts as a prompt, or clue, which is a big boost to our memory.

4. *First letter associations let us know when we're done.* When you have a first letter association for a list, you know that if you match an item or word with every letter on that list you're finished. In other words, everything you need to remember is in that first letter association.

Now you can see why the First Letter Association Technique is so useful and so popular. Let's try a first letter association exercise using the list from the Link Technique exercise:

table
pen
locket
umbrella
salt

To apply the First Letter Association Technique, I take all the first letters of the items on this list:

t p l u s

Next, I see if I can make up a word to help me remember these letters. "T-PLUS" is a rather obvious choice here. Another possible first letter association for this list might be "PLUST." When I later need to remember this list, I simply need to remember "T-PLUS" to jog my memory for table, pen, locket, umbrella, salt.

Of course, there are some drawbacks to the First Letter Association Technique. First letter associations require a bit of creative energy. In addition, these associations can be difficult to create in certain circumstances, such as when you have a list that has no words beginning with a vowel (try this with your next grocery list and you'll see what I mean). While there are ways around such problems, first letter association is not the easiest internal memory technique available. However, it possesses some unique characteristics that make it an effective way to boost your brainpower, especially if you enjoy a challenge.

### 7 The Snapshot Technique

Another great way to help yourself remember something is to picture it. We tend to underutilize our visual memory even though it is a powerful way for us to learn and recall information. The Snapshot Technique lets us take advantage of our visual potential. Simply come up with a visual picture for the information you are trying to remember. No need to get a complicated story line going—just picture what you need to recall, as if you were taking a snapshot of it. Let's try this technique on the following word list:

walk

patch

clown

fox

fair

I can help myself remember this list by picturing each of these items in my mind's eye. For "walk," I could "see" a sidewalk. "Patch" brings up the image of a patch on a pair of jeans. A clown is easy to picture, as is a fox. Finally, "fair" calls to mind the image of a county fair. By using the Snapshot Technique, I am paying closer attention to the material I am trying to learn. I am also making the information more meaningful by connecting it to a visual image.

The Snapshot Technique is one of the easiest internal memory techniques. Many people find that picturing information they are trying to learn is a simple and quick way of boosting their brainpower.

## 8 The Movie Technique

We can also use our visual advantage by making up movies, or visual associations, for things we are trying to remember. Think of this method as the storytelling technique with pictures. The Movie Technique works best if the movies:

- *Are vividly "seen."* The clearer the image for the movie is in your mind's eye, the more likely you are to remember it.

- *Have motion.* A visual association involving some kind of movement will be easier to recall.

- *Are exaggerated or silly.* Something that is unusual or funny captures our attention and is easier to remember.

Let's try the Movie Technique using the same word list we used for the Snapshot Technique:

walk

patch

clown

fox

fair

Now picture the following: A *clown* with *patch*ed clothes is *walk*ing his pet *fox* through the county *fair*grounds. Close your eyes and get a really good picture of this in your mind's eye. This visual association is vivid, has motion, and is certainly silly. You will now be able to remember this list by "seeing" this funny image.

And there you have it—eight great ways you can remember information "by head." Perhaps you've found one that you already use. The two sets of Memorcises that follow will help you figure out which technique works best for you and will give you practice using it. Remember that internal memory techniques are an important part of overall memory fitness. They can be lots of fun to use, so pick your favorite and start training your brain.

---

### Practice Your Internal Memory Technique

Need an easy and unpressured opportunity to hone your favorite technique? Here are some of my favorite things to practice on. Next time you come across one, take the chance to try out your new internal memory technique.

| | |
|:---:|:---:|
| Recipes | Directions |
| License plate numbers | Phone numbers |
| E-mail addresses | To-do lists |
| PIN numbers | Credit card numbers |

## ■ STEP 5: QUIZ ■

*This quiz will help you see how well you did with your brain training. Answer
the following questions "true" or "false" (answers appear on page 148).*

**T   F**   1. The best way to remember something is to use a complicated technique to memorize it.

**T   F**   2. Internal memory techniques work because they help give meaning to information I'm trying to remember.

**T   F**   3. There is only one internal memory technique that really works.

**T   F**   4. If I master an internal memory technique, I won't have to worry about other aspects of my memory health.

**T   F**   5. The Connection Technique involves making a connection between something I am trying to remember and something that I already know.

**T   F**   6. Repeating information to myself is no substitute for a good internal memory technique.

**T   F**   7. "ASAP" is an example of a first letter association.

**T   F**   8. Getting a mental picture of information is an effective way of improving my ability to recall it later.

**T   F**   9. The Storytelling Technique involves telling someone a story about what I am trying to remember.

**T   F**  10. Using an internal memory technique that works for me is one of the ways I can maximize my memory fitness.

## ■ STEP 5: ANSWERS ■

1. **False.** *The best way to remember something varies. This step includes eight ways to remember information. The best way to remember something "by head" is to make a habit of using a simple internal memory technique that suits your personality and lifestyle.*

2. **True.** *This is, in essence, exactly how all internal memory techniques work.*

3. **False.** *Again, there are many memory techniques available for you to use. What is important is to find the one that works for you and get into the routine of using it.*

4. **False.** *You can master all these techniques and still have lowered memory potential because you aren't taking good care of yourself. A good memory is the result of total memory fitness, not just internal memory techniques.*

5. **True.** *You can make information more meaningful and therefore more memorable by connecting it to something that you already know.*

6. **False.** *Repeating information to yourself is a very effective internal memory technique, one I call the Repetition Technique. This technique is very powerful yet so simple that many people who use it don't even feel that they are doing something to help themselves remember better.*

7. **True.** *"ASAP" is a commonly used first letter association for "as soon as possible."*

8. **True.** *Visualization is a powerful way to give information additional meaning.*

**9. False.** *The Storytelling Technique requires you to weave a story involving the information you want to recall at a later time. Of course, you may find yourself telling stories about how well you can remember using this technique!*

**10. True.** *Using an internal memory technique can play an important role in making the most of your memory.*

■ STEP 5: MEMORCISES ■

*Internal Memory Technique Exercises: Set 1*

*Use each of the techniques reviewed in this chapter to learn and remember the following information.*

1. You're teaching your eighth-grade English class the different tenses of verbs. You need to come up with a way to help your students remember them.

**VERB TENSES**
**infinitive**
**simple**
**present participle**
**past tense**
**past participle**
**future**

2. You are going to run some errands, and you realize you don't have a pocket to carry your to-do list in. You decide to try to memorize it instead.

**TO-DO LIST**
**pick up shoes at shoemaker**
**return videotape**
**buy steaks at butcher's**
**get baby present for Sally**
**deposit paycheck at bank**

**3.** It's your turn to be class parent for your fourth-grader's class, and you've prepared a presentation on butterflies. You want to remember the stages in the life cycle of a butterfly in case you're asked, so you need to find a way to memorize them.

### LIFE STAGES OF A BUTTERFLY
**egg**
**caterpillar**
**pupa**
**adult**

**4.** It's trivia night at the senior center, and you want to be on top of your game. You know one of the topics is going to be favorite children's films, and you'd like to be able to remember the names of the seven dwarfs from *Snow White*. Try each method to help yourself remember them.

### SEVEN DWARFS FROM *SNOW WHITE*
**Doc**
**Grumpy**
**Sneezy**
**Sleepy**
**Bashful**
**Happy**
**Dopey**

5. Your eight-year-old daughter has just told you that she's never heard of the Beatles. Aghast, you take it upon yourself to immediately teach her the names of the fabulous foursome. Just to be safe, you want to figure out a way to help her remember them so she can teach all her friends.

### THE BEATLES
**Paul McCartney**
**John Lennon**
**Ringo Starr**
**George Harrison**

6. You need to learn Erik Erikson's eight ages of man for the midterm in your developmental psychology course. Figure out a way to remember them.

### ERIKSON'S EIGHT AGES OF MAN
**Trust *versus* Mistrust**
**Autonomy *versus* Shame and Doubt**
**Initiative *versus* Guilt**
**Industry *versus* Inferiority**
**Identity *versus* Role Confusion**
**Intimacy *versus* Isolation**
**Generativity *versus* Stagnation**
**Ego Integrity *versus* Despair**

■ STEP 5: MEMORCISES ■

*Internal Memory Technique Exercises: Set 2*

*Now you've had a chance to figure out which internal memory technique you like best. Use the following set of exercises to train yourself to use it.*

1. You are studying for an examination on human anatomy. Figure out a way to remember the ten systems of the human body.

TEN SYSTEMS OF THE HUMAN BODY
**skeletal**
**muscular**
**integumentary**
**digestive**
**circulatory**
**respiratory**
**excretory**
**nervous**
**endocrine**
**reproductive**

2. You're taking a class on architecture and need to remember the different types of Greek columns.

GREEK COLUMNS
**Doric**
**Ionic**
**Corinthian**

3. You're teaching an eighth-grade Sunday-school class and have decided that it's time for the students to learn the Seven Deadly Sins. You want to give them a good way to remember them.

### THE SEVEN DEADLY SINS
**Pride**
**Lust**
**Gluttony**
**Anger**
**Envy**
**Sloth**
**Covetousness**

4. Your eleven-year-old is studying the solar system and needs to give a report on the moons of Neptune. Teach her your method for remembering them.

### EIGHT MOONS OF NEPTUNE
**Triton**
**Nereid**
**Proteus**
**Larissa**
**Despina**
**Galatea**
**Thalassa**
**Naiad**

5. You just got a job in a jewelry store. One of the establishment's most successful items is birthstone jewelry, so you must memorize the birthstones for each month to keep this job.

### THE BIRTHSTONES OF THE MONTHS

| Month | Birthstone |
| --- | --- |
| January | garnet |
| February | amethyst |
| March | aquamarine or bloodstone |
| April | diamond |
| May | emerald |
| June | pearl or moonstone |
| July | ruby |
| August | sardonyx or peridot |
| September | sapphire |
| October | opal or tourmaline |
| November | topaz |
| December | turquoise or lapis lazuli |

6. Learning about memory improvement has left you feeling quite philosophical. You turn to Aristotle for some highbrow reading and resolve to commit to memory his ten fundamental categories by which all things in the universe can be defined.

### ARISTOTLE'S TEN CATEGORIES

**Being**

**Quantity**

**Quality**

**Relation**

**Doing**

**Suffering**

**Having**

**Position**

**Place**

**Time**

# STEP
6

# Remember What
# You Read and See

■ IN THIS STEP YOU WILL LEARN: ■

*Why We Forget What We Read and See*
*Seven Ways to Learn a List*
*How We Remember Stories*
*How to Remember Stories Better: Just SING*

Imagine the following scene: You are sitting with your spouse eating breakfast. The morning news show is on TV, and you are flipping through the day's newspaper while discussing your upcoming vacation plans. Later in the day, a customer calls to ask you about a particular story in the paper's business section that may have a negative effect on her company. You're sure that you read the piece, but for the life of you, you can't recollect exactly what it said. Embarrassed, you play along, hoping she won't notice when you appear at a loss in the conversation.

For many of us, recalling information that we read is a frustrating memory weakness that gets in our way both at work and at home.

Working with written material is an essential part of many jobs, where we need to retain what we are reading. Yet you find yourself spending time reading and rereading this information, time that you otherwise could have spent doing something else. I have found that many adults are most concerned about the problems they have in recalling written information because of their work. I am often booked by corporations specifically to train their employees how to recall what they read as a way of boosting their productivity.

We may also be concerned about our ability to remember what we read for personal reasons. Perhaps you are annoyed when you forget something you really needed from your grocery list, or feel lost when you pick up a novel you are reading because you can't remember what happened in the previous chapter. Many retirees who take my class are concerned about keeping pace in college classes or other activities they are pursuing. Marvin H. stands out as typical of these folks:

> *This gregarious, active sixty-eight-year-old came to the program after having sold his stationery business. When working, Marvin was able to retain his business inventory in his head, a talent of which he was very proud. However, he was now having trouble holding his own in a graduate history class he was auditing at a local university. Marvin was embarrassed, not to mention a bit concerned, about how hard it was for him to remember what he had read for his course. He found it very interesting, but just couldn't keep it all straight when it came time to discuss it.*

In addition, many of us are most troubled that we forget entertainment that we see, such as movies, TV shows, or plays. Have you ever panicked when you couldn't recall what happened in a movie you saw last weekend? While this kind of information is not read, it does involve recalling a story line, which in many ways is similar to remembering written material. Of course, our inability to recall what we see becomes most apparent when we are trying to tell someone else about it, making it even more embarrassing.

If you have trouble recalling what you read or see, you are not alone. Thankfully, there are many simple steps we can take to help ourselves more effectively remember what we read and see. First, though, let's get a handle on why it may be hard for us to remember the things we read or see.

## Why We Forget What We Read and See

### DISTRACTION

As you know by now, many of us forget things simply because we are unable to actively attend to information when we are getting it. This is true as well for things that we read or see. If we are not focused on something that we are reading or watching, we are not going to sufficiently acquire the information, and will not be able to have it later when we want it.

Distraction is an especially important concern in recalling information that is read or seen. When we are busy, we often try to do many things at once. Reading the newspaper, watching a TV show, or listening to the radio often happens in conjunction with other tasks, such as having a conversation, cooking a meal, or driving to work. Rarely do we give ourselves the opportunity to focus solely on the material we are reading or seeing. As you learned in Step 1, it may be harder for us to divide our attention as we grow older, so that performing multiple tasks may make it harder for us to recall information we are introduced to during those activities.

## EVERYDAY LIFE

As you learned in Step 2, many factors in our daily experience can interfere with our ability to remember effectively. We grapple constantly with lifestyle issues that may make it harder for us to effectively attend to information we are learning. Not surprisingly, these variables can make it harder for us to learn and remember information that we read or see. For example, I often read before going to bed. I know that if I am particularly tired one evening, it will be harder for me to recall what I have read than it would if I was less fatigued. Similarly, it will be harder for you to focus on what you are reading if you are preoccupied by something stressful that is happening in your life.

Many people I speak to readily identify with the effect these everyday factors can have on their ability to remember what they read or see. Leslie B., a talented woman in her early fifties, took a class with me specifically to get help with recalling written information. Recovering from chronic fatigue syndrome, Leslie found it hard to keep up with paperwork now that she was back at her job as personnel manager for a large company. Realizing the impact her illness and other lifestyle habits had on her ability to recall what she was reading helped her understand why she was having such trouble. She was able to pace herself to avoid reading important material when she was overtired.

## YOU ONLY GET IT ONCE

When you read something, be it the newspaper, a book, or a memo for work, chances are you only go over it once. The same is true for things you see, such as movies or TV shows. When this is the case, we have only one opportunity to learn the information we are getting. If we are distracted or if other factors are making it difficult for us to focus on what we are reading or seeing, we may miss our one chance to get it. Another way of understanding how this happens is to think about how you studied in high school or college. When you had to prepare for a final exam, would you read the class material once? Of course not—most likely you reviewed it several times, to ensure that you remembered it. However, you probably rarely do that for things you read today.

## YOU DON'T GIVE IT A SECOND THOUGHT

Material that we read or see can be easier to remember if we think about *how* to remember it. Chances are you rarely look for ways to help yourself remember things that you read or see. Yet you can improve your ability to recall information such as magazine articles or movie plots by applying a simple, practical memory technique to help you do so. Internal memory techniques, introduced in the previous step, can help you successfully recall information that you may only have one chance to get.

With these reasons in mind, let's look at what steps you can take to maximize your memory power for information that you read or see.

# Seven Ways to Learn a List

Lists abound in our lives. We use lists for groceries, errands, packing—you name it, chances are you can make a list for it! Here are several techniques to help you boost your memory fitness for lists. How do these methods work? They all call on the A.M. Principle: Each will get you to focus your attention and make your list meaningful.

### 1 The Write It Down Technique

This is the best way to remember a list and my favorite technique by far. Rarely do I find it necessary to commit a list to memory. If you think about it, I'm sure this is true for you as well. For example, why would you need to recall your grocery list "by head"? After all, it's going to change every few days. Under most circumstances, you can best recall what is on a list by writing that list down and taking it with you. Writing down a list, after all, gets you to really attend to it. In addition, when you transcribe a list you have another opportunity to review it. This can be a great way to learn the list. Often we just need another chance to go over information to acquire it effectively.

Of course, there may be circumstances where you need to recall a list "by head." For example, if you are making an important presentation and don't want to refer to notes, you may want to memorize a list of the main points in your talk. List techniques are also helpful when you make up a list. We are less likely to forget to put something on a list if we use a strategy when we are writing it. And, if you've used a technique when writing your list, it will be easier to remember what was on it if you leave your list behind, which can happen to even the most organized among us. Techniques we use to give the information on a list more meaning will make that list more memorable. Here are more simple and practical techniques, then, to help you train your brain to remember lists better.

## 2 The Link Technique

As we learned in Step 5, one way you can help yourself learn a list better is to link each item to another one on the list. Then, recalling one item will remind you of a second, and that one of a third, and so on. Take the following list of randomly selected words:

paper

hat

moon

river

corn

> ### *Lists and the Listless Brain*
> Do you ever worry that writing lists will make you more forget-ful or let your brain lapse into laziness? Well, relax—there is no scientific evidence that lists lead to listlessness. While we know mental activity is important to a healthy brain, for most of us the benefit of being able to remember what we need to do is far more important. There are plenty of other ways we can exer-cise our brains, including things we really enjoy, such as games, puzzles, and hobbies. It may even be that we are better off because of the stress we avoid by using a list to remind us. So rest easy—your brain won't atrophy. Write down that list!

I can link "paper" to "hat" by thinking of a hat made of paper. Next, I connect "hat" to "moon," perhaps by imagining a crescent-shaped hat. "Moon" is easily related to "river" when I think of the song "Moon River." Finally, I can link "river" to "corn" by imagining corn growing by a river (perhaps you envision a river of corn). Now, when I recall "paper," it will remind me of "hat." "Hat" will then prompt the word "moon," "moon" will bring up "river," and so on. By linking this list, I have taken otherwise unrelated words and put them in a meaningful context that will make it easier for me to recall them later. The Link Technique is especially helpful when items naturally remind you of each other. I often use this method if I want to remember a list of points for a presentation.

### 3  The Chunking Technique
It's easier for us to recall several shorter lists than one long one. If you have a long list of items you want to remember, it will be eas-ier to do so by breaking it into several shorter ones. Many people find that this method is especially helpful with numbers. Often if

we use familiar number patterns—such as a phone number or social security number pattern—to chunk a list of digits, it will be easier for us to recall them. Let's say, for example, that you want to memorize your checking account number, which follows:

4  5  3  2  7  1  0  9  7  2

That account number will be easier for you to learn if you break it into smaller groupings, such as:

45  32  71  09  72

Since your account number has ten digits, you could also chunk it as a phone number:

(453) 271–0972

## 4  The Category Technique

In categorization, we break up the list into meaningful groups of items with labels. When we categorize a list, we are using the organization that is already inherent to that list to give it meaning. Categorization is actually one of the most powerful techniques we can use in learning a list. First, it allows us to use chunking. Second, when we use categories, we have labels for each grouping. These labels act as hints or clues for the items we are trying to remember. Using categories gives us an advantage, since it is always easier for us to recall something when we have help in doing so.

Many lists we use regularly lend themselves to being categorized. For example, grocery list items can easily be grouped into categories such as produce, dairy, baked goods, and so on. The same is true for many other common lists, such as to-do lists and packing lists. The categories you use are up to you. You may break a packing list into types of items you need, such as undergarments, shirts, slacks, and toiletries. My husband prepares a packing list by each day of travel. A seventy-five-year-old student of mine preferred to divide his packing list into where he kept items, so his categories were closet, bureau, and so on.

### 5 The Storytelling Technique

Storytelling, a technique also discussed in Step 5, is a wonderful way to recall a list. If you weave the items on the list into a story line, they will be easier to remember later. Many people like to use this kind of verbal association to give items on a list meaning that they wouldn't otherwise have. Telling a story is a great way to remember a list of things you need to do, such as errands. Let's say you had to run the following errands:

**call Mary**
**buy pet food at pet store**
**get stamps at post office**
**pick up dry cleaning**

You could help yourself remember this list by weaving the following tale: "I picked up the phone to call Mary. Then, I went right over to the pet store and found the food I needed for Spot. Next stop was the post office, where they had new stamps in. In the end, I picked up my dry cleaning and carried it home."

While any story will do the trick, you will be more likely to recall a story that is funny and exaggerated. Take the words on the list we used on page 162. A gentleman in a recent class made up the following story: "I looked pretty silly in the river by the cornfield wearing a paper hat and drinking moonshine." What a great story—I know I'll never forget it!

**6** **The Snapshot Technique**

As you know from Step 5, we can often help ourselves remember information better by visualizing it. Our visual memory tends to be strong and gives us another way to give meaning to the list. We can use this visual advantage by simply picturing in our mind's eye the items we need to remember. Take again the list from page 162, only this time try to envision each of the items as you read them:

paper

hat

moon

river

corn

By picturing each item, you are more actively attending to it and are making it more meaningful.

**7** **The Movie Technique**

You can also make up a movie to help recall a list. As you learned in Step 5, the Movie Technique will work best if it is vivid, has motion, and is exaggerated or silly. My student's story, described above, works well as a visual association: Can't you just see yourself standing in the river by the cornfield, wearing a paper hat and drinking moonshine? You could even remember a to-do list in this way. One of my most inventive students, Stella T., came up with the following movie for the same errand list we used above: "Mary is with a dog, the dog is covered in stamps, and the dry cleaner is pulling the stamps off the dog." Whatever the information you need to recall, using your visual strengths to give the items more meaning by "seeing" them is a great way to maximize your memory.

These seven methods for training your brain to retain lists more effectively are simple to use. Even if you agree that writing down a list is the best way to retain it, it's important to figure out which of the other habits for remembering a list you would like to have under your belt in case you need it. That way, you can practice this technique and be ready to use it when necessary. So, decide for yourself which of these techniques suits you best and get in the habit of using it. I guarantee you will remember lists better if you do.

## How We Remember Stories

Stories, like lists, are something most of us encounter daily. We read newspapers, magazines, memos, reports, and books. We see movies, plays, and TV shows. We may listen to stories on tape or on the radio. Most people are more concerned when they have trouble remembering a story that they read or saw than they are when they forget a list. How can we remember stories better? First, let's consider what the story is with stories.

• **Stories are organized.** One of the most important things to recognize about stories is that they have organizational structure. Every story, no matter how long or short, how simple or complicated, has a hierarchy: a main (or most important) point and the other parts of the story line, which, while they may be important, vary in their significance to the central theme. In other words, all parts of a story are not created equal. How can we figure out a story's organization? Let's look at the following short story:

> Max vacations on a lake in Minnesota during the winter, where he enjoys ice fishing and hunting. Last winter, two teenagers fell through the ice while fishing. The weather was warm and the ice on the lake had thinned. A man was nearby and pulled them out with ropes he had in his truck. Fortunately, the boys were not injured, just wet and cold.

What is the organization of this story? What is the main point? It may be easier to decipher the story's hierarchy by looking at it phrase by phrase. The chart on page 169 breaks up the story by phrase. As you read the story this time, look at how important each phrase is to the central theme, based on the rating given in the chart.

This time around, you probably got a better sense of which phrases are most important to the story line and which are incidental details. The main point of this story is that two teenagers fell through the ice. After all, the story isn't about Max's winter pleasures, but about what happened to those boys—why they were on the lake, why they fell in, how they got out, and what was the result of their mishap. That Max winters in Minnesota, or that he enjoys ice fishing and hunting, is simply not relevant to the main theme of this story. While other aspects of the story are important, such as that the boys were not injured, these details are not the most essential point of the tale. After all, if they hadn't fallen through the ice, would you be concerned about whether or not they were hurt? As we will see shortly, being able to recognize the organization of a story, no matter what that story is, will help you remember it better.

• **We get the gist**. Let's say you were discussing with a friend a movie you'd seen recently. He was trying to decide whether or not to go to see it, and you were describing what it was about. How would you do that? Would you summarize for him in a few sentences what the movie is about? Or would you recite the movie for him word for word? We do not naturally recall stories word for word. When we remember a story, we focus on the gist or heart of the story. The gist of the story is an elaboration of the main point and includes the most important aspects of the narrative. If I

| PHRASE | RATING | | | |
|---|---|---|---|---|
| | not important | somewhat important | important | very important |
| Max vacations | x | | | |
| on a lake in Minnesota | x | | | |
| during the winter | x | | | |
| where he enjoys ice fishing and hunting | x | | | |
| Last winter | x | | | |
| two teenagers fell through the ice | | | | x |
| while fishing | | x | | |
| The weather was warm | | x | | |
| and the ice on the lake had thinned | | | x | |
| A man was nearby | | | x | |
| and pulled them out with ropes | | | x | |
| he had in his truck | x | | | |
| Fortunately | x | | | |
| the boys were not injured | | | x | |
| just wet and cold | x | | | |

wanted to tell you about the story described earlier in "Winters in Minnesota," I'd say, "Did you hear what happened? Two teenagers fell through the ice, but a guy was there and pulled them out with ropes. Thank goodness they weren't hurt."

Many of us are actually used to getting the main point of a story presented separately. For example, newspaper articles are traditionally written with the most important facts of a story in the first paragraph. The headline usually summarizes the story, too. Similarly, abstracts in science journals summarize the findings reported in articles, and businesspeople receive executive summaries with long reports or business plans. Why is this practice so widespread? Because it makes it easier for us to get the gist of what we are reading.

## How to Remember Stories Better: Just SING

Now that we know what the story is with stories, how can we use this to our advantage? The answer is simple. When you want to remember a story, just SING:

**S top.** When you are finished reading or watching something you wish to remember, stop for a moment. That will give you an opportunity to focus your attention more actively on the task at hand. By pausing, you are making yourself aware that you need to concentrate. So, at the end of an article or during the movie credits, just stop and give yourself the chance to focus.

**I dentify the main point.** Next, think about the hierarchical structure of the story and find the main point. The main point is the story's backbone. All other aspects of the story revolve around it. By identifying the main point, you will be using the organization of the story to help you focus on what's important to remember.

**N ever mind the details.** Distinguishing the main point will help you determine which parts of the story are really just details. Don't sweat the details. You will remember the story better if you zero in on the main point. It's much easier to recall a story when you can build outward from its backbone, rather than trying to reconstruct it with a few details.

### *Who Wrote That Book?*
### *And Other Things We Want to Remember*

Has the name of a book, an author, a movie, or an actor slipped your mind recently? It happens to many of us. Why? Most likely because we aren't really getting that information in the first place. Think about it: When you pick up a new book, chances are you look at the cover, with the title and author's name. However, once you're deep into that novel, you don't even glance at the cover anymore, but turn quickly to where you left off so you can get back to your reading. When you do that, unless the book's title or author's name is connected to the story, you're not getting an opportunity to focus your attention on or review that title and that name. That's why later you can recall everything about the story and nothing about the title and author. Solution? When you pick up the book, make a conscious effort to focus your attention and rehearse the title and author's name. You should get and remember it rather quickly after that.

**G** et the gist. If you focus on learning the gist of a story you will remember it more effectively. Perhaps think of how you would compose the first paragraph of a news article about the story, or an executive summary of what happened in the plot. And don't worry—you'll be more likely to recollect the story's details if you work from the central theme of the story than if you begin with those details themselves.

By following these four simple steps, you can boost your brainpower for stories that you read or see. Let's try this technique with the following excerpt taken from a story in the July 1997 issue of *Automotive Engineering*:

### SINGAPORE LIMITS ITS VEHICLE POPULATION

Singapore has limited its vehicle population under a certificate of entitlement (COE) scheme that applies to vehicles purchased or built since 1990. The number of right-hand-drive cars on the road is strictly controlled and, with an exception for diplomats, no left-hand-drive cars are allowed.

The COE scheme involves a monthly auction for the privilege of owning and driving a motor vehicle that carries a COE good for 10 years. The COE is not carried by the driver, but the vehicle and whoever owns it. After 10 years, the vehicle is either scrapped or sold to countries such as India, Pakistan, and Myanmar (Burma), which are seeking used vehicles.

The total price of owning a medium passenger car amounts to between $150,000 and $200,000 (U.S.). A COE alone ranges from $32,000 to $35,000 (U.S.). In addition, there is the base price of the vehicle, plus taxes, and an import duty of 45% (based on the invoice of the vehicle and a percentage of add-on charges for insurance, freight, and custom duty on imported cars). Other charges include a registration fee of 150% of the market value or invoice price of the car and flat fees of $1,000 for a private car and $5,000 for a company car. There is also a road tax that ranges from 70 cents to $1.75 per cm$^3$ of engine displacement per year.[7]

Now, let's SING. First, stop. Focus on what you just read. Let go of distraction. Next, identify the story's main point. What is it? While the article relates some rather complex information about

---

[7] "Singapore Limits Its Vehicle Population," *Automotive Engineering*, July 1997, p. 26.

owning a vehicle in Singapore, the backbone of the story is rather simple: Singapore is limiting its vehicle population. In fact, in this example, the main point is given to you directly in the title. Never mind the details! After all, when you want to remember the story later, what's going to be more relevant: the fact that Singapore is trying to limit the number of vehicles or the road tax of $.70 to $1.75 per cubic centimeter of engine displacement per year? Finally, get the gist. The gist of this story is that Singapore is limiting its vehicle population through a program that makes it very expensive to own a car. If you get that, you've got the story. Later, you will be able to recall this central point of "Singapore Limits Its Vehicle Population," and from there the details. So, whenever you want to remember a story that you read or see, just SING. It's a practical and easy tool that will immediately help you remember stories more effectively. Why? Because you will be more actively attentive to the story and using the meaning or organization inherent to the story to make it easier to remember. And who knows, it may even make you feel like singing.

Here's a great example of how it's easier to go from the heart of the tale to the interesting details than vice versa:

*Danny T. is a sixty-one-year-old accountant who came to my classes with his wife. During one class, I asked if anyone had recently seen a movie. Danny and his wife both raised their hands. Danny began by telling us some of the details of the movie, then sheepishly realized he couldn't quite recall what the movie was about. His wife filled us in, and we went on with the class. Danny's hand popped up again later. This time he volunteered that what I was saying was true, since he'd just remembered everything about the movie once his wife had reviewed the gist of its plot. As a details kind of guy, Danny hadn't been able to tell us the whole story.*

I hope you now realize how easy it is to maximize your memory fitness for information that you read and see. There's no question that you will remember such things better if you start practicing the habits described in this step.

## ■ STEP 6: QUIZ ■

*Here is a quiz to help you see how well you can recall what you just read. Answer the following questions "true" or "false" (answers appear on page 176):*

**T  F**  1. Writing down a list of items I need to remember will weaken my memory muscles.

**T  F**  2. I can improve my ability to recall a list of items if I link each item to another.

**T  F**  3. Factors in my everyday life can make it harder for me to remember things that I read by interfering with my ability to acquire them effectively.

**T  F**  4. We tend to recall stories word for word.

**T  F**  5. I can more effectively recall a list of points to make in a presentation if I make up a story that uses them.

**T  F**  6. All aspects of a story are equally important.

**T  F**  7. One of the reasons we tend to forget things we read is that we don't have the opportunity to go over the information more than once.

**T  F**  8. A movie is not hierarchically organized.

**T  F**  9. The title of a movie may be more difficult to recall if it is not directly related to the movie's content.

**T  F**  10. I can remember a play better if I identify the main point and focus on the gist of the plot.

■ STEP 6: ANSWERS ■

**1. False.** *Writing something down is a great way to remember it. Writing requires you to pay closer attention to the information. It also gives you an opportunity to rehearse that information, and to have it so that you can go back and look at it when you need to. There is no evidence that writing down lists will weaken your memory muscles. In fact, I believe that you'd be better off writing down your list and getting your memory workout elsewhere, since it's rarely worth the aggravation of forgetting something on that list!*

**2. True.** *This is the definition of the link method described in this lesson.*

**3. True.** *Factors in our everyday lives such as fatigue, anxiety, or stress can lower our concentration, which can make it more difficult to acquire all kinds of information we want to remember, including things that we read.*

**4. False.** *We tend to recall the gist of stories rather than every word.*

**5. True.** *Using this technique, otherwise known as storytelling, makes it easier to learn and remember the points you want to make in your presentation.*

**6. False.** *Stories are hierarchically organized, with some aspects being more important than others.*

**7. True.** *We often don't rehearse information that we read on a day-to-day basis, which may make it harder for us to effectively acquire the gist of what we are reading.*

**8. False.** *A movie plot, like a story, is hierarchically organized. We can use the hierarchical organization inherent to a movie to make it easier to remember.*

**9. True.** *It is harder to recall a title, be it of a movie, book, or play, if it is not directly related to its story line. This is because we may not have enough opportunity to rehearse the title, especially when we are focused on the content of the story.*

**10. True.** *By attending to the main point and gist of a play, we will remember the play more effectively.*

■ STEP 6: MEMORCISES ■

**1.** Use the list techniques reviewed in this step to learn and remember the words on this "Practice Word List."

| | |
|---|---|
| telephone | dog |
| envelope | staple |
| frame | ring |
| level | ant |
| muffin | swing |
| garage | elm |
| park | blue |
| surface | grapes |
| heart | pasta |
| album | box |

**2.** Practice learning the numbers below using the techniques for remembering a list taught in Step 6.

694827659

39584

1048275235

9839472

**3.** Try the "Grocery List" exercise to help you practice categorizing a list.

## Grocery List, Part 1

*Here is a list of grocery items you need to buy. Read this list once and then turn to page 180.*

| | |
|---|---|
| mushrooms | club soda |
| butter | corn |
| baking soda | lemons |
| oatmeal | wild rice |
| flour | cola |
| avocado | orange juice |
| sour cream | yogurt |
| ginger ale | lettuce |
| salt | cottage cheese |
| mozzarella | lemonade |

## *Grocery List, Part 2*

*Now, write down as many items as you can
from the grocery list on page 179.*

_____   _____   _____   _____

_____   _____   _____   _____

_____   _____   _____   _____

_____   _____   _____   _____

_____   _____   _____   _____

How many did you remember?

# Grocery List, Part 3

*Here are the grocery items again. This time,*
*group the items into the categories below.*

| | |
|---|---|
| mushrooms | club soda |
| butter | corn |
| baking soda | lemons |
| oatmeal | wild rice |
| flour | cola |
| avocado | orange juice |
| sour cream | yogurt |
| ginger ale | lettuce |
| salt | cottage cheese |
| mozzarella | lemonade |

PRODUCE        DAIRY        BEVERAGES        OTHER

_____   _____   _____   _____

_____   _____   _____   _____

_____   _____   _____   _____

_____   _____   _____   _____

## Grocery List, Part 4

*Now let's see how many of those grocery items you
can recall using categorization!*

PRODUCE          DAIRY          BEVERAGES          OTHER

_____     _____     _____     _____

_____     _____     _____     _____

_____     _____     _____     _____

_____     _____     _____     _____

_____     _____     _____     _____

How did you do? Chances are you remembered more of those
items this time around. While working with this list did give you
more opportunity to learn the shopping items, categorizing them
helped you remember them better than if you had simply read
the list several times.

**4.** Begin practicing your favorite list technique on lists that you commonly use, such as your grocery list, to-do list, or packing list.

**5.** Tomorrow, recall *in writing* the story "Singapore Limits Its Vehicle Population" from page 172 (without looking at the book, of course). Then check and see how well you remembered it.

**6.** This week, practice SINGing stories while reading your morning newspaper. When you reach the end of a story, take a moment to SING. By the end of the week you'll see how much better you are able to remember what you are reading.

# STEP
## 7

# Remember the People You Meet

■ **IN THIS STEP YOU WILL LEARN:** ■

*How We Learn Names*
*Tips for Remembering Names Better*
*Seven Memory Techniques to Rev Up Your Recall for Names*

Do you have trouble remembering names? If you are concerned about your memory for names, you are not alone. In fact, forgetting names is the leading memory complaint of American adults. Students often tell me they come to my classes because they really want to remember names better. Some people tell me that they never have been able to remember names effectively, while others have noticed that they have more difficulty recalling names now that they're older. William C., a fifty-two-year-old retired auto worker and union activist, was very distressed when he began to have trouble remembering names, especially since his ability to do so had always been a point of pride for him, as it was a very important part of his union work. He could no longer go into a room with dozens of people and recall all their names as well as he could before. While most of the time people can muddle through when they forget a name, there are times when forgetting someone's name can be downright mortifying. Here are some of my favorite war stories from the name front:

> *I was introducing my new son-in-law to someone and couldn't pull up his name. Needless to say my daughter wasn't very happy with me.* —Dave W., sixty-nine-year-old musician

> *I sat next to a woman at a dinner party and talked to her the whole evening. I realized that I hadn't really listened when our hostess introduced us, but figured I'd get her name sometime when someone else used it. Well, that never happened. The next day, we ran into each other on the street and made plans to get together. I couldn't bring myself to admit that I couldn't remember her name until we'd gotten together several times. Thank goodness she could laugh about it, too!* —Susan G., sixty-three-year-old writer

> *I'd now like to introduce Dr. Cynthia Cohen . . . I mean Green!* —Anonymous forty-nine-year-old employee assistance coordinator

People will also go to tremendous lengths to hide the fact that they've forgotten someone's name. One of the best stories I've heard was about a prominent social activist and fundraiser who, when at a function and unable to remember the name of the person with whom she was speaking, would call someone else over, start to introduce them, and then pretend to drop something so she could bend down and listen as they introduced themselves to each other. I guess you could call it a variation on name-dropping!

*I Can't Place Your Face . . .*

Which happens to you more frequently: forgetting a name or forgetting a face? If you are like most of us, it's probably the name. After all, isn't it because we remember someone's face that we know we've forgotten their name? It's the rare occasion when you can't recall the name *or* face of someone you've met. This step focuses on remembering names, since that is what we experience trouble with most of the time. And of course the most likely explanation for forgetting someone's name and face is that you weren't paying attention to their name *or* to their looks when you met them.

It's always interesting to see how difficult social situations such as these are handled in other cultures. In Japan, I noticed that people always exchanged business cards at the beginning of a meeting, rather than at the end as we traditionally do here. My host explained to me that since in Japanese culture one of the worst things you can do is cause someone embarrassment, business cards are exchanged before a conversation begins, to save anyone from being in the position of forgetting a name. I found that to be very civilized and thoughtful, and try to do that myself now as often as possible.

Of course, we all *can* learn new names. Think for a moment of all the new people you've met over the past year: new colleagues, a child's friends, new neighbors. Chances are you've learned many of their names. Since names are like any other information we must remember, can we learn and remember names more effectively? Absolutely. In this lesson, we will review how we learn names and faces and some simple steps we can take to better remember the people we meet.

### How Did They Do That?

Ever had the experience of running into someone you've met once before who recalls your name, even though you don't have the vaguest recollection of theirs? Often we're left feeling a bit embarrassed and wondering how they remember so well. Chances are your acquaintance—consciously or not—is practicing a memory technique to help them remember names. While it may be as simple as really focusing on a name when they hear it, people who are great at names just have good habits when it comes to learning them. This is especially true for those individuals whose living depends on knowing people's names, such as politicians and salespersons. See if they use any of the tools I explain in this lesson on you. And you too can leave others amazed at your ability to recall their names simply by using the techniques presented here.

## How We Learn Names

In general, we learn names in the same way we learn all information:

• *We pay attention.* In order to learn someone's name, we have to be paying attention to their name when we meet them. As we learned in Step 1, in order for us to effectively remember something, we must first focus our attention on it so we can acquire it. The same is true here: We learn a name most effectively when we concentrate at the time we are first learning it.

• *We practice the name.* We also learn names when we have the chance to rehearse them. Practice, as we all know, makes perfect.

The more we hear, see, or use a name, the more likely we are going to be to recall it later. A great example of this is the names of people who are in the news. Some of them we learn (perhaps unwittingly), while others we do not:

- *What is the name of President Clinton's daughter?*
- *What is the name of the head of the Palestine Liberation Organization?*
- *What was the name of Ross Perot's running mate in the 1996 campaign?*
- *What are the names of the two winners of the 1996 Nobel Prize in Physiology or Medicine?*

How did you do? Chances are you were able to easily name Chelsea Clinton and Yasir Arafat, but had some difficulty recalling that Pat Choate was Ross Perot's vice presidential candidate and that Drs. Peter Doherty and Rolf Zinkernagel were honored with that prestigious award in 1996. Why? Because you've had more exposure to the first two names than the others, since they have been in the media more frequently. Simply because you've had more opportunity to practice them, you can recall them more effectively.

## Tips for Remembering Names Better

Why, then, do we forget names? Most of us do not always use good memory habits in learning someone's name. Let's look at some general ways we can start using right now to note names more effectively.

• *Pay attention.* If you want to remember someone's name, pay attention when you hear it. As you know by now, if you don't catch information when it's first presented to you, you have very little chance of having it later when you need it. If you are aware and make the effort to focus on a name you want to learn, you will be more likely to acquire it. If while you are being introduced to someone at a neighborhood barbecue, you are thinking about how hungry you are and how much you'd like to get to the food, you probably are not going to remember her name when you run into her on the street two weeks later. But will you have forgotten her name? No. Because you were distracted by your growling stomach, you wouldn't have learned her name initially.

---

### ■ HOT TIP ■
#### *Remembrance of Names Past*

Often we have trouble in situations that require us to recall the names of people we haven't seen in quite a while. Since we don't tap this information regularly, it can be harder to remember someone's name in the few seconds we need it. Here's a helpful tip: If you want to be a hit at your high-school reunion or family get-together, take some time before the big event to rehearse the names of the people you are likely to see there. Old picture albums or yearbooks can be a great way to remind yourself exactly who is who. It can also be a lot of fun to play a name trivia game with your spouse just before a big family event (especially if the gathering is being held by your spouse's side of the family).

---

It's also important to make sure you are making the most of your senses. Make sure you hear the name. After all, how can you possibly learn and remember something you never got to begin with? If you didn't hear the name clearly, politely ask the person to repeat it. If you are too embarrassed to take this easy step, keep in mind how much more flustered you will be when you can't remember that person's name later.

Factors in our everyday life that lower our memory potential by making it harder for us to focus our attention can also play a role in how well we learn and remember names. If you are tired, ill, or have had a few glasses of wine, you may not be able to optimally focus your attention on someone's name. Similarly, you are more prone to being distracted when you are anxious, depressed, or under stress. Some people become so anxious about remembering a name that they distract themselves and become their own worst obstacle.

*Sonia L., a sixty-two-year-old businesswoman, attended my memory seminar specifically because she had such a difficult time remembering names. She was finding that while she'd never been great with names, this problem had gotten worse for her over the past several years, and was now making her worry about her memory in general. In our class on names, she became aware of how nervous she was when meeting someone. She said her inner dialogue went something like this: "Oh, no, how am I going to remember her name? I'm never going to be able to remember it—see that, look, I've already forgotten it. I can't believe how bad my memory is. There must be something really wrong with me." Sonia later reported that she immediately had an easier time remembering names simply by realizing how much her own anxiety got in her way and by getting herself to relax in those situations so that she could focus on the task at hand.*

So, if you want to boost your brainpower for names, realize that the first step is to make the most of your attention.

---

### Getting a Name When You Didn't

Ever find yourself in a situation where you should know someone's name and you don't? Who hasn't! Here are some tips on how to get a name when you really need it:

- *Let's Make a Deal*. Make the following deal with your spouse or a friend: If either of you is ever in conversation with someone and you don't introduce them, it's because you can't remember the person's name. So, your friend or partner should introduce him or herself, thereby getting the "nameless" person to give his or her name. This presents you with a chance to get it once again. You can then say something like, "Oh, I'm so sorry, this is my (husband/wife/friend)." Just be sure you're paying attention this time around!

- *Play Cards*. Ask the person for his or her business card. This may not work in every situation, but you can't beat it when it does. Why? You get to take the card with you, giving you ample opportunity to practice the name later.

- *Do the Right Thing*. You can always just ask the person to remind you. Chances are he or she has forgotten names in the past as well—maybe even yours!

• **Be picky.** Do you think you have to remember everyone you meet? And that if you can't, you have a real problem? I certainly hope not! For example, you probably don't need to know the name of your waiter or of the checkout person at the supermarket. We all make choices every day about names we want to remember and those we don't really care about. And that's okay. On the whole, it pays to be finicky and try to remember just those names you really need to know. Of course, it can be helpful to remember names you don't really need to know. After all, everyone loves to be remembered by name; it's flattering.

Often it can be fun to practice learning names you really don't need to remember as a way of sharpening your technique. I work on my name technique whenever I take a taxicab. Recently, I had the unusual experience of getting into the same cab twice in one day. It took me the whole ride back to my office to convince the driver that he had picked me up earlier! He was shocked that I remembered him.

If you decide (consciously or not) that you aren't going to make the effort to learn someone's name, don't get upset with yourself when you can't recollect it one month later when you see them again.

• **Practice a memory habit that works for you.** Using a good memory habit for remembering names will force you to pay closer attention when you get the name. It will also help you give meaning to the name, which will make it more memorable. Following are seven habits that apply the A.M. Principle and will do just that.

Does a memory habit for promoting name recall need to be hard to learn and cumbersome to use? Of course not. A simple technique that you can easily master will work just fine. The trick is to make whatever technique you use a routine, something you do after a while without even having to think about it.

# Seven Memory Techniques to Rev Up Your Recall for Names

Let's review seven techniques to foster memory fitness for names. Keep in mind that you have to find only one that suits your personality and lifestyle. Once you've figured out which technique you're most comfortable with, all you need to do is make sure you use it.

**1** **The Repetition Technique (aka the Everyperson Method)**
If you want to learn someone's name, simply repeat it until you've learned it. You can do this silently to yourself during conversation, or use the name when speaking to the person (a close variation of the Practice Technique, discussed next). If you do nothing else but get in the habit of repeating someone's name, you will be focusing your attention on the name and giving yourself more opportunity to acquire it. This technique can also be very helpful when speaking with someone, such as a business contact, on the phone. You can write down the person's name and repeat it to yourself during the phone call, thereby increasing your chances of recalling it later—something I often do. I call the Repetition Technique the "Everyperson Method" because it's a habit that's easy for anyone to use to make remembering names easier.

**2** **The Practice Technique**
The Practice Technique boosts your brainpower for names in a very straightforward way: When you want to learn someone's name, you practice the name in specific ways during the course of your initial conversation with that person. We are more likely to acquire information we practice, since in doing so we give ourselves more opportunity to learn it. This technique is very similar to the Rep-

etition Technique, except it provides us with a very specific structure for using the name in the initial conversation. The Practice Technique has four basic steps:

- *Spell it.* Spell the name, either to yourself or out loud. Spelling the name forces you to pay closer attention to it, get it correctly, and practice it.

- *Make a comment about it.* Make a remark about the name. Making a comment about someone's name also allows you to connect the name to something or someone you already know, which makes their name more memorable. If you just think for a moment, there's always something you can say about someone's name, even if it is just, "Oh, Euripides, that's such an unusual name." Of course, make sure you say something nice about the person's name, since nothing will make *you* more memorable than making a less than kind observation about someone's name.

- *Use it first.* Use the name at the beginning of the conversation. Again, this will force you to pay closer attention and give you another opportunity to practice the name.

- *Use it last.* A simple "Well, ———, it was very nice to meet you" is a great way to end the conversation. This step will give you a final chance to rehearse the name.

These four easy steps help you learn the name more effectively merely by giving you the chance to practice it. Sometimes clients who like this technique will say they feel funny using someone's name so much in conversation. If you feel that way, you can easily modify the Practice Technique so that you do some steps silently to yourself, or skip some altogether. Even with some modification, the Practice Technique will help rev up your recall for names.

### 3 The Connection Technique

Another way to improve your recall of names is to make a connection between the name and something that is already familiar. Many of us naturally learn new information by linking it to previously learned material. For example, if someone's name is Noah, you might say or think, "Oh, as in the ark?" The Connection Technique has the advantage of being relatively quick and simple to perform, and it makes names more meaningful and memorable. Often, you can work your connection into the conversation, giving yourself an additional chance to practice the name.

### 4 The Snapshot Technique

Visualization is a powerful tool we can use to improve our recall of names. Many of us are not aware of the strength of our visual memory, yet it is usually much easier for us to recall what we see than what we hear. As I mentioned earlier, this is in part why we may forget a name but rarely forget a face. By using the Snapshot Technique, you can take advantage of the strengths you already possess in visual memory simply by picturing the person's name. When you "see" a name, you are making the abstract information, or the name, more tangible and meaningful.

Many names can easily be pictured. We are all familiar with names that are colors (Green, Brown, Black, White, Gray), that derive from jobs (Taylor, Tanner, Gardener, Shepard), or that sound like animal names (Fox, Robbins, Veale). And many names are derived from foreign languages, and you may know their meaning in that tongue. For example, I often use in my classes an exercise that includes the last name of Ehrlich. My clients who speak Ger-

*Seeing the Name: Using the Visual Advantage*

Use this fun exercise to practice your visualization skills. Read the first column of names to yourself. Next, write down as many as you can remember on a separate piece of paper. Then read the second column of names, only this time *picture* the names after you read them. Again, write down as many as you can recall.

| | |
|---|---|
| **Robin Winters** | **Candy Foote** |
| **John Bloomgarten** | **Savannah Korn** |
| **Lily Fields** | **Rose Sinder** |
| **Mark Pitt** | **Pearl Thorne** |
| **Brooke Stein** | **Glenn Spear** |

How did you do? I bet you remembered more names the second time around. Chances are what helped you the most was using your visual advantage.

man immediately "see" the person with this name as an "honest man," the direct translation of the name. While we may not be able to use the Snapshot Technique for every name, it is a quick and powerful means of capturing strengths we already have to make names easier to remember.

### 5 The Storytelling Technique

If something is unusual or extraordinary, it is more meaningful to us and therefore easier to remember. We can make a name more memorable by creating a funny or exaggerated association for it. Making up a story, or verbal association, for a name can make it easier to remember. For example, you could make a story for the name "Frank Hill" by saying to yourself, "Frankly, he's getting over the hill." As discussed in Step 5, storytelling is a method that comes naturally to many of us. While it does involve a bit more energy, storytelling is a great tool that really works.

### 6 The Movie Technique

An association can be either verbal or visual. As we learned in Step 5, the Movie Technique involves a visual association that is exaggerated and/or silly, has motion in it, and is something we can see vividly. For example, if you wanted to remember the name Earl Brickman, you could picture an earl, dressed in robes, laying bricks. While this technique may take more effort, it is very effective. By forcing you to pay closer attention and give your own meaning to the name, the Movie Technique allows you to give the name your own unique touch. Also, like the Picture Technique, it gives you the opportunity to use your visual memory advantage. If you like a creative challenge, this may be the technique for you.

### 7 The Visual Link Technique

The Visual Link Technique has the distinct advantage of letting us use something we are bound to remember—the person's face or appearance—with something we want to remember—their name. There are many things about someone's physical appearance we can "hook" their name to: We might select their forehead (high, wide, narrow), eyes (small, large, wide apart, close set), nose (roman, aquiline, small), or some other facial feature. They may be short, tall, thin, fair, ruddy . . . the possibilities are endless. Then, form a link in your mind between the feature you have chosen and the person's name. The more extraordinary and ridiculous you make the link, the more memorable it will be. How does the Visual Link Technique work? Let's say, for example, you meet a gentleman named Alfred Turnball. In looking for something about his

■ **HOT TIP** ■
*The Name Game*

Bored at a party? Get everyone to play the Name Game. See how many ways you can come up with to remember each other's names. It's fun and, let's face it, it's a useful way to get to know each other.

appearance to which you can link his name, you notice that Mr. Turnball has a particularly round chin. So you imagine his chin as a ball turning (if you have really mastered this technique you might even imagine two guys, Al and Fred, turning that ball on his chin). The next time you see Mr. Turnball, you will recognize his face, and his chin will "link" you to his name.

While the Visual Link Technique does not come easily to everyone, students I've had who can use this particular method really love it. For example, one student reported meeting a very tall and thin gentleman at a party whose name was Allen Reidy. He was able to form a connection between this person's physique and his name. Of course, you should be careful that your link uses something long-lasting about the person's appearance and that your chosen detail is not one that will change, such as clothing. And don't make the mistake of my student Ted G., who shared the following story about "missing links" in class:

*Ted G., a sixty-nine-year-old attorney, and his friends had taken to remembering a certain farmer in their neighborhood as "alarmer farmer," since the gentleman in question tended to speak in a loud, booming voice. Unfortunately, this link did nothing to help them remember the farmer's name, since it referred to his occupation instead. We couldn't even help Ted think of a better link in class, as he had no idea at all of the fellow's name!*

The Visual Link Technique, like the Storytelling and Movie Techniques, requires imagination and some effort. However, if you like this technique and adopt it as your memory habit for names, it will become easier to do with practice.

What, then, can you do to remember names more effectively? First, you can pay attention when you initially meet someone whose name you want to remember. Next, you can use a simple memory technique to help you give the name meaning and for further opportunity to practice the name. Choose the technique that best suits *you*. Believe me, a technique won't work for you if you don't like it or can't find the time to do it. You may even find that your memory technique for names blends the ones I've described above. That's great. In fact, I really enjoy hearing from students how they've personalized these techniques to maximize their effectiveness. An art dealer in my class found that connecting people's names to famous paintings helped her. There is no one right way to boost your brainpower. Whatever helps you is what you should be doing. What is most important is that you find something that works for you and then *make a habit of doing it*. If you follow these steps, you will maximize your memory effectiveness and be able to master the names of the people you meet.

### *Names to Practice On*

Try remembering the names of people you meet in the course of your day whose names you *don't* have to remember. It's a terrific way to hone your name recall technique in a nonpressured situation. Great names to practice on include those of:

your waiter or waitress
the checkout person at the grocery store
a salesclerk
an airline reservationist
your bus driver
other people's secretaries

▪ STEP 7: QUIZ ▪

*This quiz will help you see how much you've learned about remembering names. Answer the following questions "true" or "false" (answers appear on page 202).*

**T F** 1. I should try to remember the names of everyone I meet.

**T F** 2. If I can "see" a name, I'll be more likely to remember it.

**T F** 3. I am more likely to forget a face than a name.

**T F** 4. The Practice Technique helps me learn a person's name by giving me more opportunities to practice it during the course of conversation.

**T F** 5. Paying attention is not an important part of learning names.

**T F** 6. I can remember a name better if I connect it with something or someone I already know.

**T F** 7. It can be harder for me to learn a name I wish to remember if I'm anxious about being able to learn the name.

**T F** 8. The Visual Link Technique refers to picturing the person's eyes as cuff links.

**T F** 9. In order to remember names more effectively, I must master all the techniques taught in this lesson.

**T F** 10. Having a few drinks at a cocktail party may make it harder for me to learn the names of people I am meeting there for the first time.

■ STEP 7: ANSWERS ■

**1. False.** *There is no reason why you should need to remember the names of everyone you meet. In fact, we are all naturally selective about the names we try to learn for later recall. Let's face it, sometimes you barely attempt to get someone's name because you don't think it's important to remember. What's important is to use good memory habits to learn the names of people we want to remember . . . and to realize that there may be times we don't remember someone's name simply because we didn't try to learn it in the first place.*

**2. True.** *Using the Snapshot Technique, which involves "seeing" the name you are trying to learn, is a quick and powerful way to give the name additional meaning.*

**3. False.** *You are much more likely to forget a name than a face.*

**4. True.** *The steps of the Practice Technique give you four chances to practice the person's name in your initial conversation.*

**5. False.** *By now you know that attention is an essential part of learning and remembering any information!*

**6. True.** *Making a connection between something you are learning, such as a new name, and something you already know makes it more meaningful and memorable.*

**7. True.** *Anxiety is one of the many elements in daily life that can interfere with attention and concentration, thereby lowering memory potential. If this happens to you, try to relax.*

**8. False.** *The Visual Link Technique involves linking a person's name to something about their physical appearance. (Although this could be true if the person's name was Cuffe Linkes!)*

**9. False.** *Please find just one technique that works for you. Trying to master all of them will make it less likely that you'll develop the habit of using a technique that's right for you. Developing your own technique that combines those I've described is fine, of course — as long as you have one thing that you always do when you have to remember a name.*

**10. True.** *Alcohol interferes with our ability to learn new information. Does that mean you shouldn't drink? Of course not. But it does mean that you need to make choices about having a drink and being at your best for learning a new acquaintance's name.*

## ■ STEP 7: MEMORCISES ■

**1.** Practice the techniques described in this step to help you learn and remember the following names:

**Fred Lovett**
**Susan Klapper**
**Nicole Coyne**
**Lolly Mitchell**
**Steven Kimmel**
**Chris Barnes**

**2.** Start thinking about which technique you prefer. Use the "Name Worksheet" exercise on pages 205 and 206 to help you perfect your memory habit for names. On the first worksheet you are given both names and faces. The second worksheet presents only the faces, so you can quiz yourself on the names.

**3.** You can make additional name worksheets on your own. Cut several small photographs out of a newspaper and glue them to a separate piece of paper. Then photocopy the sheet of paper so you have several copies. On one sheet, write the names of the individuals under their photographs. The other sheets should include only the photographs *without* the names. You can then study the names and faces on the first sheet and use the additional sheets to test your name recall. It's a great way to continue practicing your memory habit in an unpressured way.

## ■ STEP 7: NAME WORKSHEET 1 ■

*Use your favorite technique for improving name recall to learn the names of the people pictured below.*

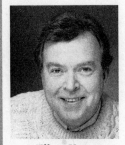

Elliot Keye

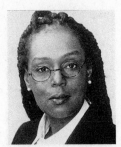

Sylvia Manchester

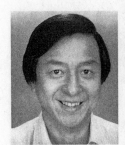

Harry Carosi

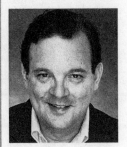

Jonah Ahl

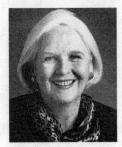

Pamela Bernard

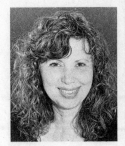

Toni Liliberte

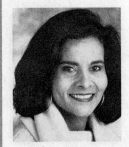

Robin Ramirez

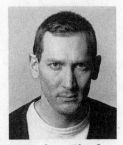

Zachary Sharf

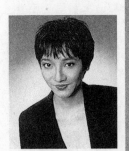

Donna Hartz

## ■ STEP 7: NAME WORKSHEET 2 ■

*Here are the same faces, but this time without the names. Use this worksheet to see how well you can remember the names of the people pictured.*

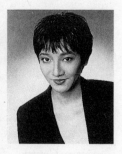

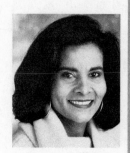

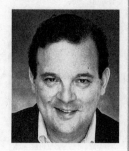

_____

_____

_____

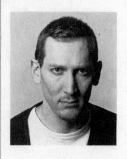

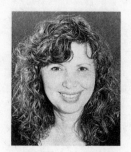

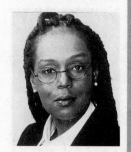

_____

_____

_____

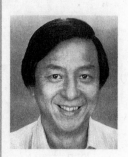

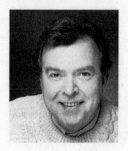

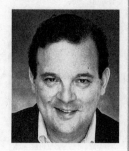

_____

_____

_____

**4.** Think of five people you've met recently whose names you'd like to remember. Write them down below. Next, come up with a way of remembering them more effectively by applying your favorite memory technique.

| Name | Technique |
| --- | --- |
| _____ | _____ |
| _____ | _____ |
| _____ | _____ |
| _____ | _____ |
| _____ | _____ |

# STEP
## 8

# Total Memory
# Maintenance

---

**■ IN THIS STEP YOU WILL LEARN: ■**

*What You Absolutely Must Remember from Each Step*
*Tips for Maintaining Your Maximum Memory Fitness*

---

By now you have had time to think about how each of the steps applies to you personally. Many of you will have already started to change your daily memory habits to help boost your brainpower. Perhaps you are paying closer attention when you want to remember something. Maybe you've turned in your old appointment book and are having fun with a new electronic organizer. Possibly you're getting into the habit of picturing someone's name when you first hear it. You are already feeling better about how well you can remember. And you know that as you continue to practice better memory habits you *will* remember better. You are on your way to maximum memory fitness.

What next? One of the most difficult things for people who have gone through a wellness program like this is to maintain the new skills they have learned as time goes on. This may sound familiar to any of you who have ever been on a weight-loss program. While you're on the diet, you may lose enough weight to get down to your goal. Yet the farther away you get from the actual time when you committed to the diet, the harder it becomes to adhere to its rules, and slowly the weight comes back. I sometimes speak with former students who experience the same thing with memory wellness. They still realize the power of better memory fitness, and they still want to remember better. They've just become lax in their memory habits.

This final step in the workout is devoted to helping you learn how you can maintain maximum memory fitness long after you have finished this book. First, let's review the most important points from each of the previous steps. Then we'll talk about your best bets for keeping your memory healthy and fit.

## What You Absolutely Must Remember from Each Step

While it is theoretically possible to memorize everything you've learned in this book, doing so would *definitely* result in information overload. Besides, you always have the book to refer to again, so why bother? What you must remember are the most central points from each step. Here's a summary:

### STEP 1: MEET YOUR MEMORY

*The A.M. Principle.* If you remember nothing else from this lesson, remember the A.M. Principle, which reminds us of the two most important steps we can take to boost our brainpower: paying *attention* and giving *meaning* to information we want to recall. I explained in Step 1 that the A.M. Principle is the backbone of this entire program. Now you understand why this is my program's golden rule.

## STEP 2: THE LIFESTYLE CONNECTION

*Lifestyle matters.* The most important point from this lesson should be easy to keep in mind, since you have daily evidence of its significance. If we want to remember better, we must take good care of ourselves, both physically and mentally. We cannot achieve better memory fitness without being aware of our overall well-being and how stress, diet, medications, and more can affect our memory potential.

## STEP 3: FOOD FOR THOUGHTS

*Diet matters.* Don't forget that a healthy diet is essential to a healthy memory. Eating well is part of taking good care of yourself, which in turn is important to remembering better. And keep in mind that supplements are no cure for an unhealthy lifestyle and poor memory habits.

## STEP 4: GET ORGANIZED

*Be organized.* Organized people remember more effectively, because being organized makes the information we need to remember more manageable. Use good organizational tools, and use them well, to maximize your memory power.

## STEP 5: TRAIN YOUR BRAIN

***Get an internal memory habit and use it.*** Get into the habit of using a simple memory technique to give meaning to information you want to remember "by head." Again, it doesn't matter which technique you choose—different people will prefer different ways of remembering, in the same way they prefer different automobiles or desserts. What's important is that you find the internal memory technique you like best and use it.

## STEP 6: REMEMBER WHAT YOU READ AND SEE

***SING.*** The best way to remember a story is to SING it: Stop, Identify the main point, Never mind the details, Get the gist. (Notice, this is what we are doing now as we summarize each step.) While we also went over how to recall lists in this lesson, I stand by my first recommendation: Write them down.

## STEP 7: REMEMBER THE PEOPLE YOU MEET

***Get a name-memory habit and use it.*** The best way to deal with America's number one memory complaint is this: Figure out which of the seven memory techniques you prefer for revving up your name recall, and then get into the habit of using it.

If you focus on these basic rules of maximum memory fitness, you will always remember how to make the most of your memory.

# Tips for Maintaining Your Maximum Memory Fitness

Now that you know what you absolutely must remember from the previous steps, let's look at the best ways to preserve the memory gains you've made through this program. Here's how you can continue to benefit from the lessons you've learned:

• *Make sure that better memory habits are part of your daily routine.*

As I often tell my students, I can *tell* you what to do to make the most of your memory power, but I can't *do* it for you. You are the only one who can integrate memory wellness into your life. The good news is that doing so doesn't have to be difficult. At first it may take a bit of effort to begin working better memory habits into your regular routine. Yet doing so will quickly become more automatic and easier. After a short time, you'll find that you don't even need to think about practicing better memory habits—you'll just do them.

• *Refresh your memory.*

What if you find that you've become rusty on recalling names or that your system of organization has fallen apart? From time to time you may feel you've slipped in a particular area of memory. Or perhaps there's a topic here you didn't really focus on your first time through that now is causing you concern. What can you do? Simply go back to the appropriate step and do it over again. The steps are designed to be used independently, as you need them. There's no reason why you can't do all the steps several times. You may even discover something new that you'd like to try. Returning for review is a great way to ensure continued memory fitness.

• *Beware the changes of life.*

When your life changes, so do the demands on your memory. Any significant life change—a new baby, an illness, a promotion, a divorce, your retirement—requires you to shift how you manage from day to day. Perhaps the life event you've experienced is stressful and you're distracted by it. Maybe you find you're not really using your memory tools because they don't really suit your new situation.

If you notice changes in your memory at the same time you're experiencing a life change, don't be discouraged. Keep in mind that such events can affect your memory. Use what you've learned here to help you reassess what now may be making it harder for you to remember. If you have trouble figuring out where the problem lies, try keeping a "forgetting notebook" for a few days (see "The Forgetting Notebook" box on page 214). Then come back to the lessons here to help you change your memory habits to better fit your new situation.

• *Be positive about your memory.*

Above all else, be positive about your memory. We will never do well at something we don't believe we can do. Consider a professional baseball player: If that player is convinced he'll hit out of the ballpark every time he's at bat, if he knows he can run circles around everyone else on the field, if he's certain he can catch anything that comes his way, he'll play his best game. On the other hand, if he's certain he'll strike out, believes he's slow as molasses, and isn't crazy about his catching, he probably won't do as well. The same is true for you. Negative thinking can lower your memory potential in just the same way it can lower an athlete's performance. In fact, some memory researchers have suggested that the real problem for older adults isn't that they can't remember, but that they *think* they can't remember.

### *The Forgetting Notebook*

If you feel your memory habits are slipping, it may be due to a lifestyle change. If you know exactly what you need to review, it's easy to open this book to the right lesson and get started. But what if you're not sure where to start? You can help yourself figure out where to begin by keeping a "forgetting notebook." Over a few days, record in a small notebook each memory mishap. For each lapse, note the following:

- *When.* Write down the time of your memory lapse.
- *Where.* Witness where you were when you forgot.
- *What.* Now's your chance to record what it was you didn't remember.
- *Why.* Using all you've learned here, think about why you forgot. You now know that you probably forgot because of something that you did or didn't do. By figuring that out, you'll be able to determine what is getting in your way on memory lane.

After a few days of keeping this forgetting notebook, review it. Look first at *why* you've been forgetting. In most cases, this in itself will tell you what's lowering your memory potential. Then look through the rest of the record. You'll definitely know where to get started once you've done so. A forgetting notebook is a great way to help you get back on the track to maximum memory fitness.

If you want to remember better you first must believe that you can. Thinking that you can't remember is a self-fulfilling prophecy. I have seen so many people who don't remember well in part because they simply don't believe that they can. You have a great deal of control over how well you remember. The steps in this book have shown you how to better exercise that power over your memory ability. Always remember that memory is part of your overall health, and as such is something you can take responsibility for and improve.

If you use these tips as you go forward from here, you will without a doubt continue on the path to a healthier memory. Here's wishing you maximum memory fitness!

■  STEP 8: QUIZ  ■

*This quiz is more like a final exam that tests your overall recall from all the lessons. Answer the following questions "true" or "false" (answers appear on page 218).*

**T  F**  1. The only way to remember better is to use a complicated mnemonics system.

**T  F**  2. Believing I can remember better will help me to do so.

**T  F**  3. If I expect to really maximize my memory, I must memorize all of the techniques taught in this book.

**T  F**  4. If I master an internal memory technique, I won't have to worry about other aspects of my memory health.

**T  F**  5. Researchers have found that persons over seventy-five cannot benefit from memory training.

**T  F**  6. Repeating information to myself is no substitute for a good internal memory technique.

**T  F**  7. Certain medications may unintentionally interfere with memory performance.

**T  F**  8. There are several dietary supplements that have been proven to boost memory performance.

**T  F**  9. I will remember someone's name better if I pay attention when I first hear it.

**T  F** 10. I can maximize my memory fitness by making better memory habits part of my everyday life.

■   STEP 8: ANSWERS   ■

1. **False.** *Remembering better is the result of better memory fitness. You can achieve better memory fitness by using better memory habits. While such habits may include internal memory techniques, they aren't limited to them. If you only use a complicated memory system and do nothing about the other issues that can affect your memory health, chances are you still won't remember more effectively.*

2. **True.** *Research suggests that our memory self-efficacy, or how well we believe we can remember, significantly affects our ability to remember.*

3. **False.** *There is no need to memorize all of the techniques taught in this book. Several different techniques are offered in each step so you can find the ones that work for you. This is because there is no single best way to improve memory. Only by figuring out the techniques that suit you personally will you actually use them to their fullest benefit. So please don't memorize them all — just find the ones that work for you and do those.*

4. **False.** *Just using an internal memory technique isn't enough. If you need to be reminded why, see the answer to the first question, above.*

5. **False.** *Research has shown that healthy adults of any age can learn new memory skills and improve their recall ability.*

6. **False.** *Repeating information to yourself is an internal memory technique, explained in Step 5.*

7. **True.** *As we learned in Step 2, certain medications may interfere with memory performance as an unintended side effect.*

**8. False.** *No nutritional supplement has been proven to improve memory performance. Despite the claims you may read on the box or label, no supplement currently on the market has met scientific standards as a safe and effective memory booster.*

**9. True.** *Paying attention to anything that you wish to remember is a necessary first step to remembering it better.*

**10. True.** *Making better memory habits part of your everyday life is the best way to get to maximum memory fitness.*

■ STEP 8: MEMORCISES ■

1. Consider how each of the things that you absolutely must remember from each lesson applies to you personally.

2. Take some time to think about how you will practice better memory habits as part of your daily life. Next, make the commitment to work those habits into your everyday routine.

# References

## Step 1: Meet Your Memory

Arenberg, D. "Comments on the Processes That Account for Memory Declines with Age." In *New Directions in Memory and Aging: Proceedings of the George A. Talland Memorial Conference.* L. W. Poon, J. L. Fozard, L. S. Cermak et al., eds. Hillsdale, N.J.: Lawrence Erlbaum Associates, 1980, 67–71.

Bureau of the Census. *Statistical Brief: Sixty-five Plus in the United States.* Washington, D.C.: Department of Commerce, Economics and Statistics Administration, May 1995.

Cerella, J. "Aging and Information Processing Rate." In *Handbook of the Psychology of Aging,* vol. 3. J. E. Birren and K. W. Schaie, eds. San Diego: Academic Press, 1990.

Craik, F. I. M., and E. Simon. "Age Differences in Memory: The Role of Attention and Depth of Processing." In *New Directions in Memory and Aging: Proceedings of the George A. Talland Memorial Conference.* L. W. Poon, J. L. Fozard, L. S. Cermak et al., eds. Hillsdale, N.J.: Lawrence Erlbaum Associates, 1980, 95–113.

Crook, T. H., R. T. Bartus, S. H. Ferris et al. "Age-Associated Memory Impairment: Proposed Diagnostic Criteria and Measures of Clinical Change." Report of a National Institute of Mental Health Workgroup. In *Developmental Neuropsychology* 2 (1986): 261–76.

Green, C. R., and K. L. Davis. "Clinical Assessment of Alzheimer's-Type Dementia and Related Disorders." In *Human Psychopharmacology,* vol. 4. I. Hindmarch and P. D. Stonier, eds. New York: John Wiley and Sons, 1993.

Hayflick, L. *How and Why We Age.* New York: Ballantine Books, 1994.

Hultsch, D. F., and R. A. Dixon. "Learning and Memory in Aging." In *Handbook of the Psychology of Aging,* vol. 3. J. E. Birren and K. W. Schaie, eds. San Diego: Academic Press, 1990.

Kinsbourne, M. "Attentional Dysfunctions and the Elderly: Theoretical Models and Research Perspectives." In *New Directions in Memory and Aging: Proceedings of the George A. Talland Memorial Conference.* L. W. Poon, J. L. Fozard, L. S. Cermak et al., eds. Hillsdale, N.J.: Lawrence Erlbaum Associates, 1980, 113–130.

Lachman, J. L., and R. Lachman. "Age and the Actualization of World Knowledge." In *New Directions in Memory and Aging: Proceedings of the George A. Talland Memorial Conference.* L. W. Poon, J. L. Fozard, L. S. Cermak et al., eds. Hillsdale, N.J.: Lawrence Erlbaum Associates, 1980, 285–311.

Lane, E., and J. Snowdon. "Memory and Dementia: A Longitudinal Survey of Suburban Elderly." In *Clinical and Abnormal Psychology.* P. Lovibond and P. Wilson, eds. New York: Elsevier Science, 1989, 365–76.

Luria, A. R. *The Mind of a Mnemonist: A Little Book About a Vast Memory.* Cambridge: Harvard University Press, 1968.

McDowd, J. M., and J. E. Birren. "Aging and Attentional Process." In *Handbook of the Psychology of Aging,* vol. 3. J. E. Birren and K. W. Schaie, eds. San Diego: Academic Press, 1990.

Miller, G. A. "The Magical Number Seven, Plus or Minus Two: Some Limits on Our Capacity for Processing Information." *Psychological Review* 63 (1956): 81–96.

Moscovitch, M. "A Neuropsychological Approach to Perception and Memory in Normal and Pathological Aging." In *Aging and Cognitive Processes: Advances in the Study of Communication and Affect,* vol. 8. F. M. Craik and S. Trehub, eds. New York: Plenum Press, 1982, 55–78.

Perlmutter, M. "An Apparent Paradox About Memory Aging." In *New Directions in Memory and Aging: Proceedings of the George A. Talland Memorial Conference.* L. W. Poon, J. L. Fozard, L. S. Cermak et al., eds. Hillsdale, N.J.: Lawrence Erlbaum Associates, 1980, 345–53.

Pogrebin, Letty Cottin. "Honey, What's Your Name Again?" *The New York Times,* 26 August 1996.

Quilter, R. E., L. M. Giambra, and P. E. Benson. "Longitudinal Age Changes in Vigilance over an Eighteen-Year Interval." *Journal of Gerontology* 38 (1983): 51–54.

Rowe, J. W., and R. L. Kahn. *Successful Aging.* New York: Pantheon Books, 1998.

Salthouse, T. "Age and Memory: Strategie for Localizing the Loss." In *New Directions in Memory and Aging: Proceedings of the George A. Talland Memorial Conference.* L. W. Poon, J. L. Fozard, L. S. Cermak et al., eds. Hillsdale, N.J.: Lawrence Erlbaum Associates, 1980, 47–65.

Sattler, J. M. "Age Effects on the Wechsler Adult Intelligence Scale — Revised Tests." *Journal of Consulting and Clinical Psychology* 30 (1982): 785–86.

Schaie, K. W. "The Seattle Longitudinal Study: A 21-Year Exploration of Psychometric Intelligence in Adulthood." In *Longitudinal Studies of Adult Psychological Development,* by K. W. Schaie. New York: Guilford Press, 1983.

Smith, A. D. "Age Differences in Encoding, Storage, and Retrieval." In *New Directions in Memory and Aging: Proceedings of the George A. Talland Memorial Conference.* L. W. Poon, J. L. Fozard, L. S. Cermak et al., eds. Hillsdale, N.J.: Lawrence Erlbaum Associates, 1980, 23–45.

Storandt, M. "Age, Ability Level, and Method of Administering and Scoring of the WAIS." *Journal of Gerontology* 34 (1979): 175–78.

West, R. L., and T. H. Crook. "Age Differences in Everyday Memory: Laboratory Analogues of Telephone Number Recall." *Psychology and Aging* 5 (1990): 520–29.

Yesavage, J. A. "Nonpharmacologic Treatments for Memory Loss with Normal Aging." *American Journal of Psychiatry* 142 (1985): 600–605.

Youngjohn, J. R., and T. H. Crook. "Stability of Everyday Memory in Age-Associated Memory Impairment: A Longitudinal Study." *Neuropsychology* 3 (1993): 406–16.

## Step 2: The Lifestyle Connection

Albert, M. S. et al. "Predictors of Cognitive Change in Older Persons: MacArthur Studies of Successful Aging." *Psychology and Aging* 10, no. 4 (1995): 578.

Barrett-Conner, E. "Rethinking Estrogen and the Brain." *Journal of the American Geriatrics Society* 46 (1998): 918–20.

Barrett-Conner, E., and D. Kritz-Silverstein. "Estrogen Replacement Therapy and Cognitive Function in Older Women." *Journal of the American Medical Association* 269, no. 20 (1993): 2637–41.

Barrett-Conner, E., and D. Kritz-Silverstein. "Gender Differences in Cognitive Function with Age: The Rancho Bernardo Study." *Journal of the American Geriatrics Society* 47 (1999): 159–64.

Benton, D., P. Y. Parker, and R. T. Donohoe. "The Supply of Glucose to the Brain and Cognitive Functioning." *Journal of the Biological Sciences* 28 (1996): 463–79.

Birge, S. J. "Is There a Role for Estrogen Replacement Therapy in the Prevention and Treatment of Dementia?" *Journal of the American Geriatrics Society* 44 (1996): 865–70.

Blazer, D., D. C. Hughes, and L. K. George. "The Epidemiology of Depression in an Elderly Community Population." *Gerontologist* 27 (1987): 281–87.

Block, R. I., and M. M. Ghoneim. "Effects of Chronic Marijuana Use on Human Cognition." *Psychopharmacology* 110 (1993): 219–28.

Blumenthal, J. A., C. F. Emery, D. J. Madden et al. "Cardiovascular and Behavioral Effects of Aerobic Exercise Training in Healthy Older Men and Women." *Journal of Gerontology: Medical Sciences* 44, no. 5 (1989): M147–57.

Breitner, J. C., B. A. Gau, K. A. Welsh et al. "Inverse Association of Anti-Inflammatory Treatments and Alzheimer's Disease: Initial Results of a Co-Twin Control Study." *Neurology* 44, no. 21 (1994): 227–32.

Bremner, J. D., J. H. Krystal, S. M. Southwick et al. "Functional Neuroanatomical Correlates of the Effects of Stress on Memory." *Journal of Traumatic Stress* 8 (1995): 527–53.

Bremner, J. D., P. Randall, T. M. Scott et al. "Deficits in Short-Term Memory in Adult Survivors of Childhood Abuse." *Psychiatry Research* 59 (1995): 97–107.

Bremner, J. D., P. Randall, T. M. Scott et al. "MRI-based Measurement of Hippocampal Volume in Patients with Combat-Related Stress Disorder." *American Journal of Psychiatry* 152, no. 7 (1995): 973–81.

Brody, J. "Relaxation Method May Aid Health." *The New York Times*, 7 August, 1996.

Brody, J. "A Cold Fact: High Stress Can Make You Sick." *The New York Times*, 12 May 1998.

Dealberto, M., N. Pajot, D. Courbon et al. "Breathing Disorders During Sleep and Cognitive Performance in an Older Community Sample: The EVA Study." *Journal of the American Geriatrics Society* 44 (1996): 1287–94.

Dey, J., A. Misra, N. G. Desai et al. "Cognitive Function in Younger Type II Diabetes." *Diabetes Care* 20, no. 1 (1997): 32–35.

Elias, P. K., R. B. D'Agostino, M. F. Elias, and P. A. Wolf. "Blood Pressure, Hypertension, and Age as Risk Factors for Poor Cognitive Performance." *Experimental Aging Research* 21, no. 4 (1995): 393–417.

Elias, P. K., M. F. Elias, R. B. D'Agostino et al. "NIDDM and Blood Pressure as Risk Factors for Poor Cognitive Performance: The Framingham Study." *Diabetes Care* 20, no. 9 (1997): 1388–95.

Etnier, J. L., W. Salazar, D. M. Landers et al. "The Influence of Physical Fitness and Exercise upon Cognitive Functioning: A Meta-Analysis." *Journal of Sport and Exercise Psychology* 19 (1997): 249–77.

Fujishima, M., S. Ibayashi, K. Fujii et al. "Cerebral Blood Flow and Brain Function in Hypertension." *Hypertension Research* 18, no. 2 (1995): 111–117.

Green, C. R., and K. L. Davis. "Clinical Assessment of Alzheimer's-Type Dementia and Related Disorders." In *Human Psychopharmacology,* vol. 4. I. Hindmarch and P. D. Stonier, eds. New York: John Wiley and Sons, 1993.

Hackman, B. W., and D. Galbraith. "Six-Month Pilot Study of Estrogen Replacement Therapy with Piperazine Oestrone Sulphate and Its Effect on Memory." *Current Medical Research Opinion* 4, supp. 3 (1977): 21–27.

Hafen, B. Q., K. J. Karren, K. J. Frandsen et al. *Mind/Body Health: The Effect of Attitudes, Emotions and Relationships.* Boston: Allyn and Bacon, 1996.

Henderson, V. W., A. Paganini-Hill, C. Emanuel et al. "Estrogen Replacement Therapy in Older Women: Comparison Between Alzheimer's Disease Cases and Nondemented Control Subjects." *Archives of Neurology* 51 (1994): 896–900.

Jenkins, M. A., P. J. Langlais, D. Delis, and R. Cohen. "Learning and Memory in Rape Victims with Posttraumatic Stress Disorder." *American Journal of Psychiatry* 155, no. 2 (1998): 278–79.

Katz, I. R., L. P. Sands, W. Bilker et al. "Identification of Medications That Cause Cognitive Impairment in Older People: The Case of Oxybutynin Chloride." *Journal of the American Geriatrics Society* 46 (1998): 8–13.

Liebman, B. "The Changing American Diet." *Nutrition Action Healthletter* 24, no. 3 (1997): 8–9.

Liebman, B. "The Fight Against Flab." *Nutrition Action Healthletter* 24, no. 10 (1997): 1–11.

Liebowitz, B. D. "Diagnosis and Treatment of Depression in Late Life." *American Journal of Geriatric Psychiatry* 4, supp. 1 (1996): S3–S6.

Maggi, S., J. A. Langlois, N. Minicuci et al. "Sleep Complaints in Community-Dwelling Older Persons: Prevalence, Associated Factors, and Reported Causes." *Journal of the American Geriatrics Society* 46 (1998): 161–68.

Mason, L. J. *Guide to Stress Reduction.* Berkeley, Calif.: Celestial Arts, 1985.

McEwen, B. S., and R. M. Sapolsky. "Stress and Cognitive Function." *Current Opinion in Neurobiology* 5 (1995): 205–16.

Meneses, A., C. Castillo, M. Ibarra, and E. Hong. "Effects of Aging and Hypertension on Learning, Memory, and Activity in Rats." *Physiology and Behavior* 60, no. 2 (1996): 341–45.

Miller, S. T., and D. A. Zapala. "Better Use of Hearing Aids in Hearing-Impaired Adults." *Journal of the American Geriatrics Society* 46 (1998): 1168–69.

Nakamura-Palacios, E. M., C. K. Caldas, A. Fiorini et al. "Deficits of Spatial Learning and Working Memory in Spontaneously Hypertensive Rats." *Behavior and Brain Research* 74, nos. 1–2 (1996): 217–27.

Neeper, S. A., F. Gomez-Pinilla, J. Choi et al. "Exercise and Brain Neurotrophins." *Nature* 373 (1995): 109.

Newman, A. B., P. L. Enright, T. A. Manolio et al. "Sleep Disturbance, Psychosocial Correlates, and Cardiovascular Disease in 5201 Older Adults: The Cardiovascular Health Study." *Journal of the American Geriatrics Society* 44 (1997): 1–7.

Ohkura, R., K. Isse, K. Akazawa et al. "Evaluation of Estrogen Treatment in Female Patients with Dementia of the Alzheimer's Type." *Journal of Endocrinology* 41, no. 4 (1994): 361–71.

Phillips, S. M., and B. B. Sherwin. "Variations in Memory Function and Sex Steroid Hormones Across the Menstrual Cycle." *Psychoneuroendocrinology* 17, no. 5 (1992): 497–506.

Pope, H. G., A. J. Gruber, and D. Yurgelun-Todd. "The Residual Neuropsychological Effects of Cannabis: The Current Status of Research." *Drug and Alcohol Dependence* 38, no. 1 (1995): 25–34.

Popelka, M. M., K. J. Cruickshanks, T. L. Wiley et al. "Low Prevalence of Hearing Aid Use Among Older Adults with Hearing Loss: The Epidemiology of Hearing Loss Study." *Journal of the American Geriatrics Society* 46 (1998): 1075–78.

Proctor, S. P., R. F. White, T. G. Robins et al. "Effect of Overtime Work on Cognitive Function in Automotive Workers." *Scandinavian Journal of Work and Environmental Health* 22 (1996): 124–32.

Ramanathan, M. "Atenolol-Induced Memory Impairment: A Case Report." *Singapore Medical Journal* 37, no. 2 (1996): 218–19.

Rowe, J. W., and R. L. Kahn. *Successful Aging*. New York: Pantheon Books, 1998.

Rozzini, R., L. Ferruci, K. Losonczy et al. "Protective Effects of Chronic NSAID Use on Cognitive Decline in Older Persons." *Journal of the American Geriatrics Society* 44 (1996): 1025–29.

Schmidt, R., F. Fazekas, M. Koch et al. "Magnetic Resonance Imaging, Cerebral Abnormalities and Neuropsychologic Test Performance in Elderly Hypertensive Subjects: A Case-Control Study." *Archives of Neurology* 52, no. 9 (1995): 905–10.

Schmidt, R., F. Fazekas et al. "Estrogen Replacement Therapy in Older Women: A Neuropsychological and Brain MRI Study." *Journal of the American Geriatrics Society* 44 (1996): 1307–13.

Sherwin, B. "Estrogen and/or Androgen Replacement Therapies and Cognitive Functioning in Surgically Menopausal Women." *Psychoneuroendocrinology* 13, no. 4 (1988): 345–57.

Sherwin, B. "Estrogen Effects on Cognition in Menopausal Women." *Neurology* 48, supp. 7 (1997): S21–S26.

Starr, J. M., L. J. Whalley, and I. J. Deary. "The Effects of Antihypertensive Treatment on Cognitive Function: Results from the HOPE Study." *Journal of the American Geriatrics Society* 44 (1996): 411–15.

Stewart, W. F., C. Kawas, M. Corrada, and E. J. Metter. "Risk of Alzheimer's Disease and Duration of NSAID Use." *Neurology* 48, no. 3 (1997): 626–32.

Strachan, M. W., I. J. Deary, F. M. Ewing, and B. M. Frier. "Is Type II Diabetes Associated with an Increased Risk of Cognitive Dysfunction? A Critical Review of Published Studies." *Diabetes Care* 20, no. 3 (1997): 438–45.

Strassburger, T. L., H. C. Lee, E. M. Daly et al. "Interactive Effects of Age and Hypertension on Volumes of Brain Structures." *Stroke* 28, no. 7 (1997): 1410–17.

Thyrum, E. T., J. A. Blumenthal, D. J. Madden, and W. Siegel. "Family History of Hypertension Influences Neurobehavioral Function in Hypertensive Patients." *Psychosomatic Medicine* 57, no. 5 (1995): 496–500.

Turner, N. et al. "Exercise Training Reversed the Age-Related Decline in Tyrosine Hydroxylase Expression." *Journal of Gerontology: Biological Sciences* 52A, no. 5 (1997): B255.

Van-Boxtel, M. P., F. Buntinx, P. J. Houx et al. "The Relation Between Morbidity and Cognitive Performance in a Normal Aging Population." *Journal of Gerontology* 53, no. 2 (1998): M147–54.

Vanhanen, M., K. Koivisto, L. Karjalainen et al. "Risk for Non-Insulin-Dependent Diabetes in the Normoglycaemic Elderly Is Associated with Impaired Cognitive Function." *Neuroreport* 8, no. 6 (1997): 1527–30.

Waldstein, S. R., C. M. Ryan, J. M. Polefrone, and S. B. Manuck. "Neuropsychological Performance of Young Men Who Vary in Familial Risk for Hypertension." *Psychosomatic Medicine* 56, no. 5 (1994): 449–56.

Waldstein, S. R., J. R. Jennings, C. M. Ryan et al. "Hypertension and Neuropsychological Performance in Men: Interactive Effects of Age." *Health Psychology* 15, no. 2 (1996): 102–9.

Weil, A. *Spontaneous Healing.* New York: Fawcett Columbine, 1995.

Wilder, L. I. *Little House in the Big Woods.* New York: Harper Trophy, 1932.

Yaffe, K., D. Grady, A. Pressman, and S. Cummings. "Serum Estrogen Levels, Cognitive Performance, and Risk of Cognitive Decline in Older Community Women." *Journal of the American Geriatrics Society* 46 (1998): 816–21.

## Step 3: Food for Thoughts

Boushey, C. J. et al. "A Quantitative Assessment of Plasma Homocysteine as a Risk Factor for Vascular Disease." *Journal of the American Medical Association* 274 (1995): 1049.

Buffington, C. K. "DHEA: Elixir of Youth or Mirror of Age?" *Journal of the American Geriatrics Society* 46 (1998): 391–92.

Carper, J. *Stop Aging Now: The Ultimate Plan for Staying Young and Reversing the Aging Process.* New York: HarperCollins, 1995.

Cassor, P. et al. "Oral DHEA in Physiologic Doses Modulates Immune Function in Postmenopausal Women." *American Journal of Obstetrics and Gynecology* 169 (1993): 1536.

Chafetz, M. D. *Smart for Life: How to Improve Your Brain Power at Any Age.* New York: Penguin Books, 1992.

Cushman, J. H. "Governors Pledge to Join Fight Against Microbe Killing Fish." *The New York Times,* 9 September 1997.

Harman, D. "Free-Radical Involvement in Aging: Pathophysiology and Therapeutic Implications." *Drugs and Aging* 3, no. 1 (1993): 60–80.

Hendrie, H. C., S. Gao, K. S. Hall et al. "The Relationship Between Alcohol Consumption, Cognitive Performance and Daily Functioning in an Urban Sample of Older Black Americans." *Journal of the American Geriatrics Society* 44, no. 10 (1996): 1158–65.

Itil, T., and D. Martorano. "Natural Substances in Psychiatry (*Ginkgo biloba* in Dementia)." *Psychopharmacology Bulletin* 31, no. 1 (1995): 147–57.

Janofsky, M. "Mid-Atlantic Seafood Industry Is Suffering." *The New York Times,* 27 September 1997, A7.

Kanowski, S., W. M. Hermann, K. Stephan et al. "Proof of Efficacy of the *Ginkgo biloba* Special Extract Egb 761 in Outpatients Suffering from Mild to Moderate Primary Degenerative Dementia of the Alzheimer's Type or Multi-Infarct Dementia." *Pharmacopsychiatry* 29 (1996): 47–56.

Khorram, O. et al. "Activation of Immune Function by Dehydroepiansdrosterone (DHEA) in Age-Advanced Men." *Journal of Gerontology* 52 A (1997): M1.

LeBars, P. L., M. M. Katz, N. Berman et al. "A Placebo-Controlled, Double-Blind, Randomized Trial of an Extract of *Ginkgo biloba* for Dementia." *Journal of the American Medical Association* 278 (1997): 1327–32.

Liebman, B. "Fruit and Vegetable Antioxidants." *Nutrition Action Healthletter*, May 1997: 14.

Liebman, B. "Vitamins and a Mineral: What to Take." *Nutrition Action Healthletter,* May 1998: 1–7.

Messier, C., and M. Gagnon. "Glucose Regulation and Cognitive Functions: Relation to Alzheimer's Disease and Diabetes." *Behavior and Brain Research* 75, nos. 1–2 (1996): 1–11.

Mezzetti, A., D. Lapenna, F. Romano et al. "Systemic Oxidative Stress and Its Relationship with Age and Illness." *Journal of the American Geriatrics Society* 44 (1996): 823–27.

Morales, A. F. et al. "Effects of Replacement Doses of DHEA in Men and Women of Advancing Age." *Journal of Clinical Endocrinology Metabolism* 78 (1994): 1360.

Penland, J. G. "Dietary Boron, Brain Function and Cognitive Performance." *Environmental Health Perspectives* 102, supp. 7 (1994): 65–72.

Perrig, W. J., P. Perrig, and H. B. Stahelin. "The Relation Between Antioxidants and Memory Performance in the Old and Very Old." *Journal of the American Geriatrics Society* 45 (1997): 718–24.

Petersen, A. "The Making of an Herbal Superstar." *The Wall Street Journal,* 24 February 1998.

Riggs, K. M. et al. "Relations of Vitamin $B_{12}$, vitamin $B_6$, Folate, and Homocysteine to Cognitive Performance in the Normative Aging Study." *American Journal for Clinical Nutrition* 63 (1996): 306.

Rowe, J. W., and R. L. Kahn. *Successful Aging.* New York: Pantheon Books, 1998.

Sano, M., C. Ernesto, R. G. Thomas et al. "A Controlled Trial of Selegiline, Alpha-tocopherol, or Both as Treatment for Alzheimer's Disease." *New England Journal of Medicine* 337, no. 8 (1997): 572–73.

Schardt, D. "Remembering Ginkgo and DHEA." *Nutrition Action Healthletter,* May 1998: 9.

Schardt, D., and S. Schmidt. "Fear of Forgetting." *Nutrition Action Healthletter,* May 1997: 3–7.

Stoppe, G., H. Sandholzer, J. Staedt et al. "Prescribing Practice with Cognitive Enhancers in Outpatient Care: Are There Differences Regarding Type of Dementia? Results of a Representative Survey in Lower Saxony, Germany." *Pharmacopsychiatry* 29 (1996): 150–55.

Tolonen, M., M. Halme, and S. Sarna. "Vitamin E and Selenium Supplementation in Geriatric Patients: A Double-Blind Preliminary Clinical Trial." *Biological Trace Element Research* 7 (1985): 161–68.

United States Department of Agriculture: Center for Nutrition Policy and Promotion. *The Food Guide Pyramid.* Home and Garden Bulletin no. 252, 1992.

## Step 4: Get Organized

Intons-Peterson, M. J., and G. L. Newsome. "External Memory Aids: Effects and Effectiveness." In *Memory Improvement: Implications for Memory Theory.* D. Herrmann, H. Weingartner, A. Searleman, and C. McEvoy, eds. New York: Springer-Verlag, 1991.

Moscovitch, M. "A Neuropsychological Approach to Perception and Memory in Normal and Pathological Aging." In *Aging and Cognitive Processes: Advances in the Study of Communication and Affect,* vol. 8. F. M. Craik and S. Trehub, eds. New York: Plenum Press, 1982, 55–78.

Murray, B. "Data Smog: Newest Culprit in Brain Drain." *American Psychological Association Monitor* 29, no. 3 (March 1998): 1.

Petro, S. J., D. Herrmann, D. Burrows et al. "Usefulness of Commercial Memory Aids as a Function of Age." *International Journal of Aging and Human Development* 33, no. 4 (1991): 295–309.

## Step 5: Train Your Brain

Boswell, J., and D. Starer. *Five Rings, Six Crises, Seven Dwarfs and 38 Ways to Win an Argument: Numerical Lists You Never Knew or Once Knew and Probably Forgot.* New York: Viking Penguin, 1990.

Johnson, O., ed. *1996 Information Please Almanac: The Ultimate Browser's Reference.* Boston: Houghton Mifflin Company, 1996.

Labouvie-Vief, G., and J. N. Gonda. "Cognitive Strategy Training and Intellectual Performance in the Elderly." *Journal of Gerontology* 31, no. 3 (1976): 327–32.

McEvoy, C. L., and J. R. Moon. "Assessment and Treatment of Everyday Memory Problems in the Elderly." In *Practical Aspects of Memory: Current Research and Issues.* M. M. Gruneberg, P. E. Morris, R. N. Sykes, eds. New York: John Wiley and Sons, 1998.

Oswald, W. D., R. Rupprecht, T. Gunzelmann et al. "The SIMA-Project: Effects of 1 Year Cognitive and Psychomotor Training on Cognitive Abilities of the Elderly." *Behavioral Brain Research* 78 (1996): 67–72.

Yesavage, J. A. "Nonpharmacologic Treatments for Memory Losses with Normal Aging." *American Journal of Psychiatry* 142 (1985): 600–605.

## Step 6: Remember What You Read and See

"Singapore Limits Its Vehicle Population." *Automotive Engineering,* July 1997: 26.

## Step 8: Total Memory Maintenance

Rowe, J. W., and R. L. Kahn. *Successful Aging.* New York: Pantheon Books, 1998.

West, R. L., L. K. Boatwright, and R. Schleser. "The Link Between Memory Performance, Self-Assessment and Affective Status." *Experimental Aging Research* 10 (1984): 197–200.

# Index

# About the Author

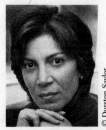

© Durston Saylor

Dr. Cynthia Green is the founding director of The Memory Enhancement Program at the Mount Sinai School of Medicine in New York City. Dr. Green teaches memory improvement in a number of settings, giving her the unique opportunity to see firsthand what people are looking for in a memory fitness program.

Dr. Green holds a Ph.D. in clinical psychology from New York University. Since 1990 she has served on the faculty of Mount Sinai Medical School and the Mount Sinai Medical Center, where she is an assistant clinical professor in the department of psychiatry. Dr. Green has worked in the field of memory for many years, serving in a variety of roles within the Mount Sinai Medical Center's Alzheimer's Disease Research Center. In addition to her command of the area of healthy memory function and memory improvement, Dr. Green's expertise includes the differential diagnosis of Alzheimer's disease and related disorders as well as functional disability in Alzheimer's disease. Dr. Green has authored several professional journals and articles, about Alzheimer's disease and related disorders. In addition, she has appeared in a number of technical videos used internationally for training in the assessment of memory disorder.

Dr. Green is also president of Memory Arts, a company that provides memory fitness training to corporate clients and organizations. She lectures widely to audiences about memory. Dr. Green lives with her family in northern New Jersey.

To learn more about the Total Memory Workout visit Dr. Green at www.totalmemory.com